Coaches Guide to
DRUGS
AND
SPORT

Kevin R. Ringhofer, PhD
Martha E. Harding
Harding, Ringhofer & Associates, Inc.

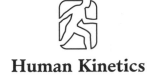

Human Kinetics

Library of Congress Cataloging-in-Publication Data

Ringhofer, Kevin R.
    Coaches guide to drugs and sport / Kevin R. Ringhofer, Martha E.
    Harding.
        p.   cm.
    Includes bibliographical references and index.
    ISBN 0-87322-715-8 (pbk.)
    1. Doping in sports.   I. Harding, Martha E.   II. Title.
    RC1230.R56   1995
    362.29'08'8796--dc20   95-16965
                                                                                      CIP

ISBN: 0-87322-715-8

Permission notices for material used from other sources appear on pp. xi-xii.

Contributing Author: Malissa Martin, EdD, ATC
Developmental Editor: Jim Kestner
Assistant Editor: Jacqueline Eaton Blakley
Editorial Assistant: Andrew Starr
Copyeditor: David Frattini
Proofreader: Bob Replinger
Indexer: Jacqueline Brownstein
Text Designer: Judy Henderson
Typesetter and Layout Artist: Kathy Boudreau-Fuoss
Photo Editor: Boyd LaFoon
Cover Designer: Jack Davis
Illustrator: Craig Ronto
Printer: Gilliland Printing, Inc.

Printed in the United States of America

10   9   8   7   6   5   4   3   2   1

Human Kinetics
P.O. Box 5076, Champaign, IL 61825-5076
1-800-747-4457
Canada:
Human Kinetics, Box 24040, Windsor, ON N8Y 4Y9
1-800-465-7301 (in Canada only)
Europe:
Human Kinetics, P.O. Box IW14, Leeds LS16 6TR, United Kingdom
(44) 1132 781708
Australia:
Human Kinetics, 2 Ingrid Street, Clapham 5062, South Australia
(08) 371 3755
New Zealand:
Human Kinetics, P.O. Box 105-231, Auckland 1
(09) 523 3462

Dedication

Coaches Guide to Drugs and Sport is dedicated to our families. Without the continued support of our spouses, Kathy and Terry, our work and this book would not be possible. Our children, Kristen, Sarah, and David, have inspired us to do our best. It is our hope that our work will make a difference for them, their friends, and other young people growing up in America.

Contents

Acknowledgments

Many people have influenced our work in preventing abuse of alcohol, tobacco, and other drugs. We are especially grateful to the following people who made key contributions to our work with coaches and ultimately to this book:

The National Federation of State High School Associations, and its current executive director, Bob Kanaby. Like his predecessor, Brice Durbin, Bob believes that school activities are more than events or contests. As the "other half of education," school activities are opportunities to help young people grow. Bob is a role model for both of us.

The National Federation TARGET program and its staff, particularly John Heeney, Susie Reineke, Lois Charley, Dick Stickle, and Kathy Perry. They made our work with their member state associations possible and have been a source of professional and personal strength.

A true innovator, Dorothy McIntyre of the Minnesota State High School League. Dorothy began in the early 1980s sponsoring and conducting prevention workshops for school administrators, activity staff, and student leaders. Her graciousness and kindness to us continues to this day.

Our many state association colleagues. Although we met through business, these people have become our friends. Over the past 10 years, we have witnessed their incredible commitment to young people and watched them make decisions based upon that commitment, often when it wasn't easy or popular to do so. Their commitment has inspired us and made our work so much more enjoyable.

Athletic directors throughout the country who share their ideas and stories and keep reminding us to make prevention practical. We particularly thank Bill Mayo, an athletic director in Blytheville, Arkansas. This loyal, encouraging, thoughtful man contributed greatly to the success of our early work as Harding, Ringhofer & Associates, Inc.

Our mentors and friends, Tom Griffin and Roger Svendsen, and our other colleagues at Hazelden, many of whom continue to work with us as associates. With them we learned approaches that could help coaches, athletic directors, and athletes prevent problems with tobacco, alcohol, and other drugs.

Finally, our editors at ASEP, Jim Kestner and Karen Partlow. Karen had the vision for this book, and Jim guided us through the development and publication of it. Also, thanks to Malissa Martin for her contributions to several chapters of this book.

Credits

Figure 1.2: Compiled from *Minnesota Student Survey, 1989-1992: Reflections of Social Change*, by Minnesota Department of Education and Risk Reduction Unit, 1992, St. Paul, MN: Minnesota Department of Education. Copyright 1992 by Minnesota Department of Education. Adapted with permission.

Tables 1.2 and 2.1: Compiled from *Athletic Participation? Students Give Their Views* [pamphlet], by Iowa High School Athletic Association, 1990, Boone, IA: Iowa High School Athletic Association. Copyright 1990 by author. Adapted with permission.

Table 3.1: From *When Is When?* [pamphlet], by K. Ringhofer and M. Harding, 1993, Minnetonka, MN: Harding, Ringhofer & Associates, Inc. Copyright 1993 by Harding, Ringhofer & Associates, Inc. Reprinted with permission.

Figures 3.2, 5.1, 7.2, 9.1, and 10.1: From *TARGET Leadership Training Manual*, by Harding, Ringhofer & Associates, Inc., 1994, Kansas City, MO: National Federation TARGET Program. Copyright 1994 by National Federation of State High School Associations TARGET Program and Harding, Ringhofer & Associates. Used with permission of National Federation of State High School Associations TARGET Program, 11724 NW Plaza Circle, P.O. Box 20626, Kansas City, MO 64195-0626, (816) 464-5400.

Figure 3.4: Reprinted with permission from "Dietary Guidelines for Americans," by U.S. Department of Agriculture and U.S. Department of Health and Human Services (Center for Substance Abuse Prevention), 1991, *Prevention Pipeline*, **4**(5), p. 68.

Figures 9.2 and 10.2: From *Student Assistance Model: The Response Component* by J. Funk, R. Svendsen, K. Cunningham, and T.M. Griffin, 1989, Center City, MN: Hazelden Foundation. Copyright 1989 by Hazelden Foundation. Reprinted with permission.

Chapter 1 opening photo: © CLEO Freelance Photo.

Chapters 2, 3, 5, 6, 10, and 11 opening photos: © Terry Wild Studio.

Chapters 4, 7, 8, and 9 opening photos: © Mary Langenfeld Photo.

Chapter 12 opening photo: © F-Stock/Brian Drake.

Introduction

We created *Coaches Guide to Drugs and Sport* as a source book of ideas for preventing problems with tobacco, alcohol, and other drugs through athletics. The overall goal of this book is to help you use your leadership position and the opportunity of athletics to convey a positive nonuse message to young people.

Coaches Guide to Drugs and Sport will help you take the following actions:

- Explain the role of athletics in reducing problems with use of tobacco, alcohol, or other drugs. You will be able to address the skepticism of other school faculty, parents, and young people about the role of athletics in prevention. You will understand your role as a coach in preventing tobacco, alcohol, and other drug use, and you will learn how your knowledge and skills as a coach can be applied to prevention. You will know how many young people are using tobacco, alcohol, and other drugs, and you will understand why some young people choose to use drugs and others do not.

- Set positive examples regarding the use and nonuse of tobacco, alcohol, and other drugs. You will learn how your attitudes and behavior set an example for young people and be able to discuss the appropriate use or nonuse of tobacco, alcohol, and other drugs with your colleagues.

- Establish and enforce rules for effective deterrence. You will explore some of the basic premises of effective rules and laws and be able to explain the rationale for rules and their consequences to young people and their parents. You will feel more prepared to enforce rules fairly and consistently and be able to work with others to write or revise, if necessary, athletic policies.

- Use formal and informal opportunities to give information about tobacco, alcohol, and other drugs. You will understand how young people receive messages that promote the use of tobacco, alcohol, and other drugs, and you will be able to use multiple opportunities to counteract these messages. You will be able to conduct preseason meetings as one method of formally reaching parents and young people, and you will be able to recognize and use informal, teachable moments throughout the season and the year.

- Use your influence to involve students and parents in prevention. You will explore many additional strategies to help prevent problems with tobacco, alcohol, and other drugs through athletics, such as student leadership training, parent networks, and parent-sponsored after-event parties. You will learn how you can be instrumental in getting parents and athletes involved, because they are often the most appropriate people to carry out these strategies.

- Respond effectively when you become concerned about a student. You will define your legitimate role in responding to athletes who are experiencing problems, including those who are using tobacco, alcohol, and other drugs. You will be better equipped to talk to athletes when you become concerned, and you will know the resources that are available to back you up.

- Identify school and community resources that can help you prevent problems, respond to troubled students, and promote healthy lifestyles. You will learn the advantages of a broadbrush, team approach to student assistance programs and understand how you can support your athletes through every step of the student assistance process. You will have resources at your fingertips which will help you evaluate and choose resources for teaching about tobacco, alcohol, and other drugs.

What You Will Not Find in These Pages

- An admonition to drop your job as coach and assume the job of prevention specialist. Although we believe you can play a very significant role in preventing alcohol, tobacco, and other drug use among young people, we recognize that this is clearly neither your primary job nor the foremost goal of sports.

- Detailed information about tobacco, alcohol, and other drugs and their effects on an athlete's performance. Our goal is not to train you to be a drug information expert. You do not need to memorize all of the names or physiological effects of various drugs to know that the use of most drugs can be harmful for a young person. The drug culture continuously changes, including the street names for various drugs. There are many sources for this information, including a reference guide to common drugs in Appendix B. While having access to these facts is helpful, it is not necessary for sending a consistent nonuse message. Most young people do not want more information about tobacco, alcohol, and other drugs. Instead, they want opportunities to talk with trusted adults about issues surrounding the use of these drugs.

- A long treatise on chemical dependency and its effects on individuals, teams, and families. A whole profession, with its own philosophy, institutions, and language, has developed to address chemical dependency. The extent of the information available on chemical dependency can be overwhelming. Although chemical dependency is a significant and devastating problem, it affects a minority of young people and adults. While treatment for chemical dependency may be necessary for some young people, it is not your job to determine which young people need treatment and which do not. Chemical dependency is only one of many problems that are created by the use of tobacco, alcohol, and other drugs. You do not need to be an expert on chemical dependency to respond to young people who use tobacco, alcohol, and other drugs, or to help prevent them from using these drugs in the first place.

- Simplistic, one-dimensional solutions. Prevention aims to reduce all types of problems connected with tobacco, alcohol, and other drugs. Effective prevention of these problems requires multiple activities over a long period of time. It is not a single event. Effective prevention is a process that requires planning and a long-term commitment from many individuals, groups, and organizations in a community. As important as we believe the role of sports in prevention to be, athletics is still just one aspect of a young person's life and one voice in a whole community.

- Overwhelming data that paints a negative picture of young people and the choices they make. The image of despair and hopelessness is the legacy of the 1980s because during that time more data became available on young people and the problems they face. While some of this data is accurate, it often is used to emphasize the negative—rather than the positive—aspects of growing up in America. *Coaches Guide to Drugs and Sport* will avoid "ain't it awful" hand wringing.

What You Will Find in These Pages

- An approach to prevention that emphasizes the positive benefits of choosing not to use tobacco, alcohol, and other drugs. This approach is based on data that shows many young people are choosing not to use these drugs and are making healthy and life-affirming choices in many areas of their lives. This approach is based on the concept of protective factors as well as risk, looking at the strengths young people and their families have rather than simply at their weaknesses.

- An affirmation of the major role that an individual coach can play in prevention. Prevention cannot—and should not—be left to the so-called "experts." We view prevention as everybody's business. When the major influences in the life of a young person are sending the same messages, the impact of these messages is extremely powerful. You are one of many messengers who can be a significant force in helping young people choose not to use tobacco, alcohol, and other drugs.

- An assessment of the assets you have at your disposal for helping young people make healthy choices. As a coach, you already have many of the important skills that can simply be translated to the prevention arena. You also have an important relationship with the young people you coach. What you do and say—as well as what you do not do or say—to young people can have a great impact upon them. Your opinion is as important—if not more so—than factual information about tobacco, alcohol, and other drugs.

- An approach that is compatible with other prevention strategies. The concepts found here enhance other school- and community-based prevention strategies. Although *Coaches Guide to Drugs and Sport* focuses on the role of the coach, most of the concepts and ideas apply to adults who sponsor or direct any cocurricular activities and to all cocurricular participants. Many concepts and ideas also apply to preventing other problems that affect young people.

- Reasonable and appropriate prevention strategies that fit into the job you are already doing. Being a prevention advocate does not require extensive training or hours of work in addition to the time you are already committing to young people and your community. Your role is to use the natural opportunities you have to help prevent problems from occurring and to refer athletes to appropriate resources when problems do occur.

As we write *Coaches Guide to Drugs and Sport*, we picture in our minds the thousands of coaches who have helped us shape and refine our ideas about the proper role of athletics in preventing tobacco, alcohol, and other drug problems. It is they who have kept us from unrealistic ideas about the capacity of athletic programs to take on this job. It is they who have demanded realistic and workable solutions to their very real concerns about actual students. It is they who have shown us, time and time again, that concerned coaches—working in tandem with other individuals and organizations—can make a tremendous difference in the choices young people make. They have sustained and reinforced our hope and vision.

At the same time, we picture also the countless young lives these coaches touch. We have listened to thousands of young people speak of these important adults in their lives and know from their stories the things they yearn for in their relationships with their coaches. Their forthright, honest questions and ideas have also challenged us to move from theoretical to practical strategies.

Beyond these students, we remember their parents, who support and encourage their involvement in athletics and otherwise powerfully shape their lives. By letting us in on their hopes and dreams for their children—and by sharing their fears and struggles as parents—they have helped us understand how they can be active partners with you in preventing use of tobacco, alcohol, and other drugs.

Scouting the Arena

Part I of *Coaches Guide to Drugs and Sport* provides a solid foundation for understanding why athletics is such a powerful arena for preventing the adolescent use of tobacco, alcohol, and other drugs.

We have had the opportunity to witness the power of this approach. After more than a decade of watching people apply the principles in *Coaches Guide to Drugs and Sport*, we are fully convinced that athletics can change community norms concerning tobacco, alcohol, and other drugs.

In the next two chapters you will read about your influence on young athletes and about how this influence extends beyond your team members into the community. You will discover how many young people are using tobacco, alcohol, and other drugs; what kinds of drugs they are using; and how young athletes are different from or similar to nonathletes. You will examine the reasons why some athletes choose to use tobacco, alcohol, and other drugs and why many others choose not to use. This information will provide a foundation for understanding the five major actions you can take to prevent the underage use of tobacco, alcohol, and other drugs.

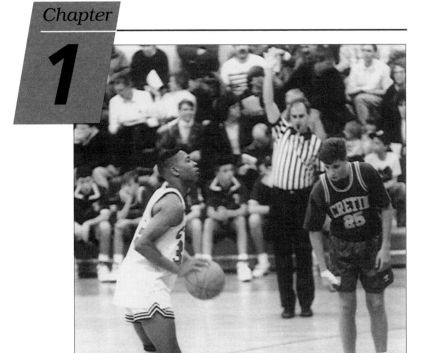

Chapter

1

The Presence of Drugs in Sport

Chapter Warm-Up

Chapter 1 will help you understand the role of athletics in reducing use of tobacco, alcohol, and other drugs. You will be able to talk to school faculty, parents, and young people about why it is important to work through athletics to prevent problems. You will know how many young people are using tobacco, alcohol, and other drugs and how athletes are similar to or different from nonathletes.

Why Athletics?

"Athletics aren't to blame for the problems young people experience, but sometimes athletics provide the kind of nurturing environment where a germ can grow."

Nancy Marshall, Gymnast

Responsibility for preventing tobacco, alcohol, and other drug-use problems often shifts from one faction of a community to another. Churches and other religious organizations are given the responsibility for preventing problems when tobacco, alcohol, and other drug-use problems are seen as a moral issue. Law enforcement personnel are charged with the responsibility of enforcing laws prohibiting use when problems are seen as a legal issue. Schools are asked to take on the responsibility for educating students about tobacco, alcohol, and other drugs when communities believe problems are caused by a lack of knowledge. When drug-use problems are seen as a societal failing, social service agencies are asked to fix the ills that originally created the problems. When we are talking about adolescent drug use, everyone looks to parents as both the cause of—and the solution for—tobacco, alcohol, and other drug-use problems.

In actuality, this is a complex and multifaceted issue, encompassing moral, legal, mental, social, physical, spiritual, and familial factors. Every organization listed above has a role to play in both preventing and responding to tobacco, alcohol, and other drug-use problems. Current prevention philosophy views prevention as everybody's business. Communities are encouraged to define their standards about tobacco, alcohol, and other drug use and to involve all segments of the community in promoting those standards.

In recent years, increasing attention has been given to athletics as an important vehicle for prevention efforts. *Coaches Guide to Drugs and Sport* is based on the premise that coaches directly influence the young athletes on their teams. It is also based on the premise that athletes and coaches influence others in the community: friends, family, and fans.

Many Young People Participate in Sports

The popularity of sports and the large number of students involved make athletics a unique and legitimate platform for prevention efforts. Across the country, almost 50% of our nation's high school students participate in school athletic programs (Extra Curricular Involvement, 1995). When you add the number of young people who participate in community athletic programs, it becomes obvious that athletics offer an opportunity to send prevention messages that simply should not be missed. For many young people, sports are a significant reason they like school, and most students believe that sports and fitness are an important part of life.

Coaches Have a Unique Relationship With Athletes

As a coach, you have a unique and powerful relationship with many young athletes. If they are interested in a sport, you often hold the key to their participation and make critical decisions about their ability to play a particular position, to compete in games, or to advance into leadership positions. Young athletes may also see you as a role model and mentor. What you say and do can influence their behavior. As a significant adult in a young person's life, you can also help balance the peer pressure they may feel. It is likely that peer pressure is not greater on young people today than it was a generation or two ago, but that peer pressure is less balanced by positive adult influences. The number of significant adults in young people's lives has diminished. Young people are more often living in single-parent homes, they are often isolated from grandparents and other relatives, and they move more often. Family size has also decreased, leaving young people with smaller extended families. All these factors make it difficult for young people to develop and maintain relationships with adults. As a result, you may be one of the few significant adults in a young person's life while also maintaining a natural connection with that young person through athletics.

Athletes Become Attached to Their Teams

Young athletes often become strongly attached to their team and to their coach. This bond is created when they experience the satisfaction of being a part of the team. The bond is strengthened as they develop and use skills which allow them to contribute to the team. It is reinforced when they receive recognition for their efforts. Recognition gives them the incentive to continue to contribute and reinforces the skills they have learned. Because of this attachment, young athletes often will emulate the standards of their team. If team members have decided not to use tobacco, alcohol, and other drugs, then an individual team member will be more likely to make the same choice. However, if influential team members choose to use, then it may be more difficult for an individual team member to abstain. Well-designed athletic programs can increase the likelihood that team members will adopt nonuse standards both during school and after school hours. Working with groups to whom young people are attached appears to be a sound prevention strategy (Hawkins & Catalano, 1992).

Sports Provide Unique Learning Situations

"Athletics are not a panacea; they are a platform."

John Heeney, National Federation TARGET Program

Opportunities to give information about tobacco, alcohol, and other drugs continually arise during the course of a season. These teachable moments happen when a sports figure is arrested for an alcohol- or drug-related offense; when advertisers link alcohol to participation in sports; when a rule is violated; when a game is won or lost; and when athletes make personal decisions—good or bad—about tobacco, alcohol, or other drugs. Because of your relationship with young athletes, you can use these times to let them know how you feel about the use of tobacco, alcohol, and other drugs. You can also teach other important skills, such as handling winning and coping with losing, dealing with the stress of competition, cooperating for a common goal, and demonstrating leadership on and off the field. The skills and values you teach through athletics can influence young people throughout life, particularly if you help them see how those skills and values apply to areas other than athletics.

Athletes Are at Risk for Tobacco, Alcohol, and Other Drug Problems

Unfortunately, young people who participate in school athletics are not immune to problems with tobacco, alcohol, and other drug use. In fact, some research shows that athletes may use alcohol at slightly higher rates than the general student population. Some of the circumstances surrounding athletics may place them at higher risk for use of other substances, such as steroids and smokeless tobacco. This chapter and chapter 2 will explore these risks and pressures in more detail.

The Public Pays Attention to Sports

Newspapers, radio stations, and television networks give extensive coverage to sports events, which both reflects the public's interest in sports and promotes ongoing attention to athletics. This public attention is a major reason for using athletics as a vehicle for prevention. Just as advertisers use athletics for selling tobacco, alcohol, and other products, concerned community members can use athletics to promote positive standards.

Athletes and Coaches Are Role Models

Because of the attention given them by fans, young athletes and their coaches are role models for the community. The choices they make about tobacco, alcohol, and other drugs can and do influence others. Their attitudes and behaviors can reach beyond their teams to others in their school or community.

Athletics Provide Access to Parents

Prevention research consistently shows that what parents do and say is a major influence on the choices their children will make about tobacco, alcohol, and other drug use, but prevention specialists have long been frustrated with their inability to involve parents in prevention. Athletics provide one of the most effective means to reach parents. Athletic events generally draw more parents than any other school-related event, providing a unique opportunity to reach this captive audience.

Taken together, these reasons create a compelling argument for using athletics as a vehicle to promote positive standards about tobacco, alcohol, and other drug use and nonuse. Indeed, because of its unparalleled access to young people and their parents, athletics can promote a wide range of healthy community standards.

The Extent of Tobacco, Alcohol, and Other Drug Use Among Athletes

"My coaches and extracurricular sponsors all have steered me to a drug- and substance-free life . . . . Being able to choose school activities over idle time and tempting behaviors has had a big impact on my life by leaving me with a stronger sense of direction and a place to turn in the face of impending danger."

Jason Butler, Silver Lake High School, Silver Lake, KS, On TARGET, May 1993

This section will give you current information about tobacco, alcohol, and other drug use and nonuse among athletes and nonathletes. Before you flip to the next chapter, we will summarize in 60 seconds four important concepts that will help you work with young people. The rest of the section will give you more in-depth information about drugs and athletics.

Here are the four most important things you need to know. Set your stopwatch:

- Alcohol is still the most widely used—and misused—drug. It does not matter which age group you are talking about—eighth graders through college students—young people use alcohol more than any other drug.

- There are more similarities than differences between athletes and nonathletes in their drug-using behavior. Unfortunately, athletics do not seem to insulate young people from tobacco, alcohol, and other drug use. The differences are interesting, however, and may indicate the type of influence athletics have on the choices young people make about drugs.

- Prevention efforts clearly make a difference. There has been a marked decline in the use of all drugs, including tobacco and alcohol, over the past decade.

- Combined efforts are more useful than single efforts. Young people who get information from both their parents and their schools tend to use less than their peers who get information from other sources, such as the media or their friends.

Here is how we can speak with conviction about these four topics. We will tell you what we know and how we know it, and we will raise some interesting questions for you to consider.

Alcohol Is Still the Most Widely Used—and Misused—Drug

By the time they are seniors in high school, about 9 in 10 students will have used alcohol (Johnston, O'Malley, & Bachman, 1994). Slightly more than half of the senior class will have used alcohol within the last 30 days. More than one quarter will have drunk to intoxication (defined as having five or more drinks in a row) at least once in the last two weeks.

Contrast these statistics with those of other drugs (Table 1.1). By the time they are seniors in high school, 4 in 10 students will have tried an illicit drug other than tobacco or alcohol. In the last 30 days, less than 2 out of 10 will have used an illicit drug. When you examine the use of any individual illicit drug other than marijuana, less than 4% of the senior class will have used it in the last 30 days.

We are not attempting to minimize the attention given to illicit drug use as a serious national problem. When nearly a fifth of a given class of students is using an illicit drug, it is cause for concern. However, in our efforts to curb the use of these drugs, we must not lose sight of the fact that alcohol and tobacco—two drugs that are legal for adults—will create more problems for people as adolescents and adults than all of the other drugs combined.

Knowing that alcohol is the most commonly used and misused drug, you can counteract parental statements such as: "I'm not so worried about my son drinking; at least he's not using drugs." And knowing that young people often share this viewpoint, you can use every opportunity to reinforce the fact that the use of alcohol and tobacco is both illegal and risky behavior for adolescents.

Table 1.1 Tobacco, Alcohol, and Other Drug Use During the Past 30 Days			
Type of Drug	8th Graders	10th Graders	12th Graders
Alcohol	26.2	41.5	51.0
Cigarettes	16.7	24.7	29.9
Smokeless Tobacco	6.6	10.4	10.7
Marijuana	5.1	10.9	15.5
Stimulants	3.6	4.3	3.7
Inhalants	5.4	3.3	2.5
Hallucinogens	1.2	1.9	2.7
Cocaine (including crack)	0.7	0.9	1.3
Tranquilizers	0.9	1.1	1.2
Steroids	0.5	0.5	0.7

Note. Thirty-day use is commonly used as an indicator of current drug use. Compiled from Johnston et al. (1994).

There Are More Similarities Than Differences Between Athletes and Nonathletes in Their Drug-Using Behavior

We used to believe that if we got young people "into sports and off the streets," they would stay away from drugs. We know now that this statement is only partly true, depending on the drug, the individual athlete, and a host of other factors. Here is a sampling of what we know about five drugs—alcohol, cigarettes, smokeless tobacco, marijuana, and steroids—and their relationship to athletics.

Alcohol

Many studies have reported that high school athletes tend to use alcohol at about the same rates as nonathletes, with some showing higher use (Carr, Kennedy, & Dimick, 1990; Skolnick, 1993). In college, athletes may become more involved in the problematic use of alcohol—drinking to intoxication more often, driving after drinking, or riding with someone who had been drinking—more often than nonathletes (Nattiv & Puffer, 1991).

Cigarettes

On the other hand, athletes are less likely to smoke cigarettes than are nonathletes. In 1991, researchers from the Center for Disease Control reviewed data on more than 11,000 9th through 12th graders and concluded that "sports participation may influence smoking behavior" (Escobedo, Marcus, Holtzman, & Giovino, 1993, p. 1391). Indeed, they found that students who participated in interscholastic sports were less likely than their noncompetitive peers to be regular or heavy smokers and that, as the number of sports played increased, the proportion of regular or heavy smokers decreased. They hypothesized that

> the lower rates of smoking for students who participate in interscholastic sports may be the result of greater self-confidence derived from such participation, additional counseling from coaching staff about smoking, reduced peer influences about smoking, perceptions about reduced sports performance because of smoking, greater awareness about the health consequences of smoking, and greater desire to present a neat and conventional appearance. Further research about the possible role that participation in sports or other extracurricular activities may play on smoking may help to identify new smoking prevention strategies. (p. 1394)

We would add a few questions to consider: Do young people who smoke decide not to participate in sports in the first place? Do athletes who smoke regularly heavily impair their performance so that they cannot compete well enough to remain on teams? Do parents of athletes smoke at a lesser degree, thus sending a more consistent message to their children about smoking? Whatever the reason, athletes smoke less than their peers.

Smokeless Tobacco

Smokeless tobacco is enjoying a resurgence of popularity in America, particularly among adolescent males. Nearly 20% of male seniors in the United States used smokeless tobacco in the last 30 days, compared to about 2% of female seniors. The use of smokeless tobacco in the past 30 days is twice as high in non–college-bound senior students and more than twice as high in rural areas (Johnston et al.,1994). If you coach boys in a rural area, you may consider providing even more emphasis on prevention of smokeless tobacco use.

Unfortunately, it appears that the correlation between reduced cigarette smoking and athletics does not hold true for smokeless tobacco. The Centers for Disease Control has found an inverse relationship: Athletes were more likely than nonathletes to use smokeless tobacco (U.S. Department of Health and Human Services, 1994).

Why is there a difference in the use of these two tobacco products by athletes? Is it because smokeless tobacco is seen and promoted as a safe alternative to smoking? Is it seen and promoted as being a part of sports? Do young males believe that smokeless tobacco is macho?

"My volleyball and basketball coach has greatly influenced me to avoid substances. She is the best friend I have in the school. She sets a good example . . . . She does not tolerate her athletes using substances . . . . This rule [gives] you another reason to remain substance free, because I do not want to jeopardize my chances of playing sports."

Cari Hassell, Maplewood HS, Nashville, TN, On TARGET, May 1993

Young athletes may be less likely to use smokeless tobacco during their season of play. According to a survey of 3,795 Iowa high school male athletes, 20% reported that they had used smokeless tobacco within the past year, with 13% reporting use during their competitive season (Iowa High School Athletic Association [IHSAA], 1990). Incidentally, this relationship also holds true for alcohol, tobacco, and, to a lesser degree, for all of the other drugs surveyed (Table 1.2). The IHSAA speculates that "the reasons for this are the well publicized negative effects these substances have on performance and the student athlete not wanting to get caught breaking the rules during the season" (p. 10).

Table 1.2 Use of Drugs In and Out of Season		
Type of Drug	Use During Past Year	Use During Season
Alcohol	45%	25%
Cigarettes	23%	12%
Smokeless Tobacco	20%	13%
Marijuana	6%	4%
Amphetamines or Speed	6%	4%
Cocaine (including crack)	3%	2%
Barbiturates or Tranquilizers	3%	2%
Steroids	4%	3%

Note. Compiled from the results of a survey of 3,795 male athletes.
Compiled from Iowa High School Athletic Association (1990).

"Our head baseball coach, who also teaches health courses, has shown his players the effects of smokeless tobacco. He won't allow us to use it on the playing field and encourages us strongly not to participate in the use of smokeless tobacco off the field. I believe that he has a great effect on all of his players."

Andrew Dixon, Rancho HS, North Las Vegas, NV, On TARGET, May 1993

Marijuana and Other Illicit Drugs

Benson (1990) found that even limited involvement in school extracurricular activities (defined as one hour or more per week in school sports, clubs, or organizations) is correlated with lesser involvement in use of illicit drugs, including marijuana.

Steroids

Only about 2% of high school students will try steroids (Johnston et al., 1994). However, use of steroids is higher among high school boys (3.5%). According to a study on male high school seniors, the main reason given for using steroids was to improve athletic performance. Young people also use steroids in an effort to improve their appearance (Buckley et al., 1988).

From these studies it is apparent that we cannot assume that young people involved in athletics are not using tobacco, alcohol, or other drugs. We can share this information with our colleagues and with our athletes' parents to help them understand the importance of working through athletics to prevent young people from using drugs.

Prevention Efforts Clearly Make a Difference

The use of all drugs, including alcohol and tobacco, reached a pinnacle in the late 1970s or early 1980s. Increased public concern, coupled with major federal and state funding of prevention efforts, began to make headway in decreasing the use of drugs other than alcohol in the mid-1980s. It was not until the late 1980s, however, that alcohol finally followed the dramatic decline seen earlier in illicit drug use. This decline in the use of all drugs continued for nearly a decade. The National Federation of State High School Association's TARGET Program was begun in 1984; it has encouraged its member associations and schools to become involved in prevention through cocurricular activities.

It is clear that when we begin to obtain a consensus about the adolescent nonuse of tobacco, alcohol, and other drugs, we can make a difference. Look at Figure 1.1. Among the senior class in the United States, the use of alcohol in the past 30 days has decreased almost 30% since its high in 1978. The use of any illicit drug dropped more than half, from a high of 38.9% in 1978 and 1979 to less than 20% in the early 1990s. Cigarette use in the last 30 days dropped to less than 30% from a high of 38.8% in 1976.

That is the good news. But now, for the bad news: As we write these pages, the major successes in prevention that we have enjoyed over the past 10 years are threatened. For the first time in nearly a decade of decline, researchers from the University of Michigan's Institute for Social Research (Johnston et al., 1994) report that the use of tobacco and many other drugs among American teenagers

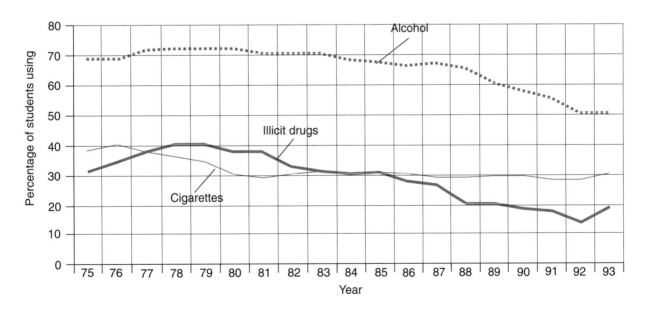

Figure 1.1 Trends in 30-day use of drugs, 1975-1993.

Note. This data examines trends in 30-day use of tobacco, alcohol, and other illicit drugs by seniors in high school. Approximately 17,000 seniors from across the country participated in this study.

Compiled from Johnston et al. (1994).

is increasing. In the results of their 19th annual survey, the investigators report a sharp rise in marijuana use throughout the country at 8th-, 10th-, and 12th-grade levels, as well as an increase in the use of stimulants, LSD, and inhalants. They also note an increase in cigarette smoking in all three grades. Two of the key attitudes that are associated with lower use—personal disapproval of use and perception of risks associated with drug use—also seem to be relaxing at all three grade levels.

We can use this information to encourage students, parents, and our colleagues to continue their vigilance. We can know with assurance that our efforts to prevent problems make a difference, and we can share this optimism with others. As we face our concern about other adolescent issues—violence, teen pregnancy, HIV, AIDS, and other sexually transmitted diseases—we need to continue our efforts to prevent tobacco, alcohol, and other drug use.

Combined Efforts Are More Useful Than Single Efforts

> "It's very easy to stay drug free when there is encouragement from someone. [My sponsor] is dedicated not only to her group, Bulldogs Against Drugs (BAD), but to her students as well. She works hard to help young people get the education they need while they lead a drug-free life."
>
> *Robyn David, Albuquerque HS, Albuquerque, NM, On TARGET, May 1993*

Recent data from nearly 100,000 teenagers have decisively shown that at least two messengers—parents and schools—are more effective than either could be alone (Minnesota Department of Education and Risk Reduction Unit, 1992). When students do not receive information about alcohol from either their parents or the school, nearly twice as many will use alcohol than their peers who receive information from both the parents and the school (Figure 1.2). It is beneficial when parents are the most important source of information—20% of

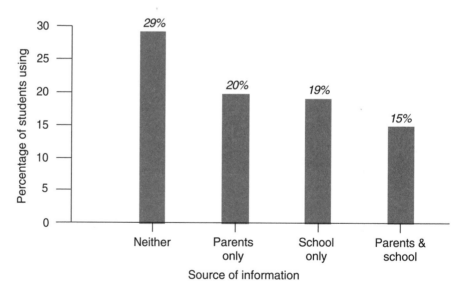

Figure 1.2 Monthly alcohol and other drug use related to primary source of information.

Note. This chart combines 6th, 9th, and 12th graders from a study of 90,000-131,000 students.

Adapted from Minnesota Department of Education and Risk Reduction Unit (1992).

these students will use alcohol, compared to 29% of students who are not getting this information from their parents. Schools make a difference, too: 19% of the students who say the school is their primary source of information will use alcohol. But when students receive information from both their parents and the school, the percentage of those who use alcohol drops to 15%—nearly half that of their peers who, presumably, get most of their information about alcohol from the media, their friends, or other sources.

We can use this information to challenge those who believe that teaching about tobacco, alcohol, and other drugs is solely the parents' job, and we can continually bolster parents' perception that they do make a difference in their children's lives. We need them to be partners with us in prevention.

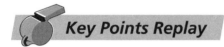 **Key Points Replay**

■ As a highly visible part of the school and community, athletics provide a unique opportunity for prevention. Because of the popularity of athletics and the visibility of coaches and athletes, prevention efforts often reach beyond teams and athletes and into the school and community.

■ As a coach, you have a special relationship with your athletes. Your influence has a significant effect on the choices your team and athletes make about tobacco, alcohol, and other drugs.

■ Alcohol is the most widely used and misused drug.

■ Athletes are not immune to tobacco, alcohol, and other drug-use problems. Many of the young people we coach have used, are using, or will use tobacco, alcohol, and other drugs.

■ Prevention efforts make a difference. The most effective prevention programs encourage many messengers to send the same message. You are one of these messengers. Working in cooperation with parents and other school- and community-based efforts, we can make a difference.

2

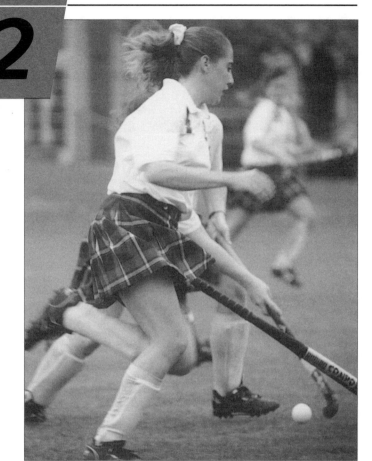

Making the Choice to Use or Not

Chapter 2 will help you understand why young athletes make the choices they do about tobacco, alcohol, and other drugs. You will explore the conditions surrounding athletics that may put some young athletes at risk for use. By understanding what motivates some athletes to use and the reasons why many choose not to use, you will be able to reduce the impact of the motivations to use and promote the positive benefits of choosing not to use.

Why Athletes Use Tobacco, Alcohol, and Other Drugs

There are many reasons why people use tobacco, alcohol, and other drugs. Drugs are prevalent in our society, and we use drugs in many different ways. Drugs are used to cure ailments, help us relax, get us going in the morning, or put us to sleep at night. Often, we want to change something about our physical, emotional, or mental state. Also, we expect that the change should happen quickly. Most of us have experience with the quick results drugs can provide.

We may believe that sports provide an opportunity for young people to be involved in a positive activity that can keep them from using tobacco, alcohol, and other drugs. We hope that their awareness of fitness and health will deter them from using these drugs. This is probably true for some athletes, but for others, sports may put them in situations which fuel their desire to use drugs for quick results. Athletes probably are motivated to use tobacco, alcohol, and other drugs in the same way as other young people, and athletes may face unique pressures.

To Experience Pleasure

Like many others who use tobacco, alcohol, and other drugs, athletes may experience pleasure when they use certain drugs. Just like some other young people, athletes may like the feelings and sensations associated with drug use and may find that drugs quickly produce these desired sensations. Drinking alcohol or smoking either cigarettes or marijuana may help an athlete relax. Cocaine may produce euphoria and more energy. Amphetamines may also provide energy and the ability to stay awake to continue in activities. Athletes may also learn to associate the use of these drugs with fun. Certain drugs, including alcohol, may help them feel less inhibited. They may find themselves having fun during activities that may make them uncomfortable when they are not using, like talking to people of the opposite sex, meeting new people, or dancing. Some activities may be risky and dangerous if a young person is under the influence of alcohol or other drugs (driving, swimming, or diving in hazardous areas are a few examples). However, because the athlete is having a good time, he or she may not think about the risks.

To Take Risks

Nattiv and Puffer (1991) discovered that collegiate athletes were more likely than nonathletes to be involved in high-risk health behaviors. Some of these high-risk health behaviors were: three or more alcoholic drinks per sitting, driving while intoxicated from alcohol or under the influence of drugs, riding with impaired drivers, not always using seat belts, not wearing helmets when riding a motor scooter or motorcycle, having three or more sexual partners per year, and not always using contraception. Nattiv and Puffer conclude that evidence from sport psychology suggests that some athletes are more likely to have a personality type that likes thrill-seeking behavior, excitement, and stimulation through physical activity. It is possible that the same quest for adventure and the same interest in defying challenges may encourage some athletes to choose other risky behaviors, including the use of tobacco, alcohol, and other drugs.

To Belong

Many young athletes have their identity wrapped up in their ability to participate in a sport. Being a part of a team often provides their most significant source of friendship and support. Athletes may use tobacco, alcohol, and other drugs to fit in with others; they may believe that drug use is an expectation within a particular group. People often emulate the standards of groups to which they are attached. If it appears that the norm of the group or the team is to drink alcohol, the athlete may also choose to drink to gain acceptance. If the norm of the group or the team is to stay straight, the athlete may choose not to use in order to be accepted.

To Be Like Their Heroes

Extensive advertising of beer on televised sporting events and the marketing of alcohol by former sports stars are only two of many examples of how sports have become an advertising vehicle for alcohol. The televised use of champagne in the locker room may also encourage the mistaken idea that teams should celebrate their victories—and drown their defeats—with alcohol. The use of smokeless tobacco on the playing field by professional athletes, their coaches, and their managers has inextricably linked chewing tobacco with athletics, particularly baseball. The public's interest in potentially performance-altering drugs, such as anabolic-androgenic steroids, has been fanned by the media, which highlights any occasion when an athlete has been banned from a sport because of steroid use. Even drug testing at the collegiate, professional, and Olympic levels contributes to the sense that good athletes can be better athletes by using these drugs. These connections may lead some athletes to believe that athletics and drugs go hand in hand.

To Cope With Stress

Many people in our society use tobacco, alcohol, and other drugs as a way to cope with stress or to escape from stressful situations. All young people face pressures and situations that are stressful and may put them at risk for problems. Competing demands from school, activities, family, friends, and work can create tremendous stress for young people. As many as 20% to 25% of adolescents live in households where alcohol and other drugs are a serious problem (Svendsen & Harding, 1987). Athletes are not protected from many of these risk factors. They may, indeed, experience a special set of risks and pressures. The following are some possible pressures for

In the Smoky Mountain Conference in the mountains of western North Carolina, Hayesville High School and Cherokee High School students use halftime at a football game to share antidrug and antidrinking messages with their communities. The students felt it important to demonstrate that the two schools could compete aggressively on the courts and playing fields and still emphasize sportsmanship and friendship.

On TARGET, February, 1993

athletes that may place them at risk to use tobacco, alcohol, and other drugs.

Visibility

Athletes are visible and vulnerable to criticism from the entire community. Athletes compete and perform in front of crowds. At some levels of competition, the media may also cover the event in the local newspaper or provide radio or television coverage. The success or failure of an individual athlete is often a highly public—not a private—matter. For some athletes, this attention is exciting and motivating. For others, it can be stressful and potentially devastating.

High Expectations

Pressure to perform, excel, and win can come from many different sources, including coaches, family, friends, fans, media, and the athlete. According to a survey of male high school athletes, two thirds of those surveyed felt there was pressure on them to win. These athletes indicated that the primary source of this pressure was their own expectations for winning. Pressure from their coach was the second strongest source, with their community and parents exerting a lesser amount of pressure to win (Table 2.1).

Table 2.1 Sources of Pressure to Win	
How many feel pressure to win?	66%
What is the source of pressure?	1. Self
	2. Coach
	3. Community
	4. Parents

Note. Compiled from the results of a survey of 3,795 male athletes.

Compiled from Iowa High School Athletic Association (1990).

Self-Expectations.   Many athletes have extremely high expectations for themselves—expectations that begin with making the team and extend to playing a particular position, excelling, and being the best player on the team or in the league. When there is a gap between the expectations that an athlete holds and actual performance, the athlete can experience depression and feelings of low self-worth. Similarly, some athletes are obsessed with, or have become accustomed to, winning. Because of a variety of factors that determine the outcome of contests, such expectations may be unrealistic and lead to frustration when the athlete or the team loses.

Expectations From Coaches.   An overemphasis on winning from coaches can exacerbate the stress that young athletes experience as they participate in sports. When only top performers are rewarded,

"Playing football or becoming class president does not ward off addiction . . . . Perhaps engaging in school activities makes a child more likely to resist trying drugs, but the danger is always present. The sure way to avoid drug problems is to avoid all use of illegal drugs, including alcohol."

Lowell Horton,
On TARGET,
March 1990

young people may conclude that winning is the only important aspect of sports. Inappropriate criticism of players or inadequate positive encouragement may make some young people feel they simply cannot measure up to a coach's expectations. When asked about their expectations of coaches, young people frequently state that they appreciate coaches who treat them as whole people, not simply as players. They want coaches who will provide positive feedback as well as constructive criticism, and they admire coaches who support them when they lose as well as when they win.

Expectations From Family, Friends, and Fans.   Parents, siblings, other family members, friends, and fans may also have high expectations for an athlete's performance on the field. The community often expects that athletes will continue to improve. If they are good as freshmen, they will be superior as seniors. One athlete commented, "A competitor of mine matured early and was a terrific athlete in his freshman year. I was only 5 feet 2 inches in 9th grade, but by 12th grade I was captain of the team. He continued to be a good athlete, but his growth and skills leveled off. The perception was that I reached my full potential as an athlete but my competitor did not."

Many times athletes also feel expectations to perform off the field. They may be expected to talk with fans and media, to attend social functions, including parties, or to speak in public. In some communities, athletes are expected to attend parties where alcohol or other drugs may be consumed. It is assumed that they will join in or be a leader in drinking alcohol or using other drugs. Fans may even buy alcoholic drinks for an athlete. It may be difficult for the athlete to turn down this gift without making a scene. As one athlete said, "When I was in college and went into a bar, people knew who I was. The bartender bought me a drink. Soon other people were buying me drinks. I thought the attention was great but didn't know how to say 'no thanks' to the alcohol without offending someone."

Erratic Time Demands

Some sports require intense preparation throughout the season and few demands in the off-season. Athletes may find it difficult to cope with these erratic time demands. Some athletes find off-season or rest periods stressful because they are unable to find activities to occupy their free time. Others feel more stress during the season when they must attempt to balance the competing demands of their sport, family, friends, and, for many, their jobs.

Separation From Family and Friends

Practice schedules, travel to contests in other communities, and fatigue that results from training and competition may draw athletes away from family, friends, and other positive relationships. These relationships often provide an essential support system for the athlete. An athlete may feel not only stress from not meeting expectations of family and friends but also a loss of support from these vital people. Intensive involvement in athletics may also preclude involvement in other beneficial areas of an athlete's life.

Role Conflicts

Characteristics like strength, size, speed, and aggressiveness may be emphasized in particular sports and, in fact, are key ingredients to excel in those sports. Using or developing these attributes may cause a conflict for some athletes. For many young female athletes the aggressive skills they develop on the playing field, along with the strong, muscular body type that is often essential to successful competition in athletics, may be in conflict with their concept of what a young woman should be. It may also be in conflict with the images and expectations that their peers—both boys and girls—hold. For some boys, the physical aggressiveness encouraged in sports like hockey or football may counter what they learn about appropriate behavior from other sources.

To Hasten Recovery

In our society, many drugs are used in an effort to alleviate or reduce the symptoms or complications of a variety of ailments. For instance, aspirin is used to get rid of a headache and antibiotics to reduce the effects of an infection. The use of drugs for therapeutic reasons is compounded by athletic injuries. Anti-inflammatory drugs may be used to reduce the swelling from an injury and speed the healing process. Pain-killing drugs may be used in an effort to speed up both the rehabilitation process and the workout schedule to get an athlete back into competition. These drugs may be used so that an athlete can compete with lesser pain that could otherwise limit or stop participation in sports.

To Improve Performance

A number of athletes use drugs to improve performance. The athlete may want this performance edge in order to produce more victories for the team, win a position over a teammate, or have the same advantage as or an even greater advantage over an opponent.

A variety of drugs have been used in the effort to improve performance in addition to the well-publicized use of anabolic-androgenic steroids. Female gymnasts may use drugs to block growth and development, because the altered center of gravity that accompanies these physical changes can be a performance disadvantage. Caffeine has been used in an attempt to give more energy and improve endurance. Cocaine has been used to increase energy. Amphetamines have been used to increase aggressiveness, and alcohol and marijuana have been used to help athletes relax prior to a contest or event.

This drive to improve performance or continue to perform at a high level is strong in many athletes. We only need to observe many of the rituals athletes perform to understand the strength of this desire. Many athletes eat certain foods prior to events, put on a uniform in a particular fashion, or adhere to a particular warm-up routine if they have experienced success after previously following these routines. One coach remarked, "Some athletes will do anything if they think it is connected with winning. If they ate spaghetti before a winning match, then they'll eat spaghetti before every game. If they think a bath helped them relax, they'll race home, hop in the tub, jump out, race back, and jump on the bus just before it pulls out, because they'll be convinced the bath helps them relax. Some won't change their socks if they think the socks bring them luck." In addition to drugs, athletes have also used vitamins, laxatives, amino acids, and blood-doping to improve performance.

To Look Better

In our society, we place great importance upon appearance. We are bombarded with advertisements from clothing, cosmetic, and related industries about how we can improve our appearance and how our appearance is linked to our success. In addition, appearance can affect performance for some athletes. Bodybuilding is clearly a sport where appearance directly affects performance. In physical contact sports, size or physique can have a profound psychological impact on an opponent. Some athletes use drugs like anabolic-androgenic steroids in an attempt to improve their appearance as well as their performance. Amphetamine use, leading to weight loss, can also be used to improve appearance.

Why Athletes Choose Not to Use Tobacco, Alcohol, and Other Drugs

If these are some of the reasons that young athletes choose to use tobacco, alcohol, and other drugs, then what is the flip side? Why do some athletes choose not to use? What reasons can we give them? Often our first response is, "Don't use tobacco, alcohol, and other drugs because they're against the law." Or we may say, "It's against the school rules" or "It's against my rules, and I'm the coach." Among young athletes across the country, rules and laws are rarely given as the most important reasons for choosing not to use. Three studies of college athletes sponsored by the National Collegiate Athletic Association (NCAA) support our observations. These studies looked at the major reasons collegiate athletes chose not to use various drugs. The fact that some drugs were illegal, that they might get caught using, or that the use of a particular drug was against the coach's rules were selected by only a small percentage of the athletes, in connection with only a few of the drugs listed (Anderson, Albrecht, & McKeagg, 1993; Anderson & McKeagg, 1985; Anderson & McKeagg, 1989).

We do not wish to minimize the importance of laws, school rules, or athletic codes of conduct. These factors set standards of behavior for high school athletes that eventually may become internalized. But we have to go beyond laws, rules, and consequences to other reasons for choosing not to use. Three studies (Anderson et al., 1993; Anderson & McKeagg, 1985; Anderson & McKeagg, 1989) report the following primary reasons that college athletes gave for not using or for stopping the use of a particular drug:

- The athlete was concerned about the health effects of the drug.
- It was against the athlete's beliefs.
- The athlete did not like the drug.
- The athlete had no desire to experience the effects of the drug.
- The athlete felt there was no need to use the drug.

High school seniors echo these reasons and add another: The athletes felt that their parents would object. According to a survey of nearly 100,000 high school students (Minnesota Department of Education and Risk Reduction Unit, 1992), these were the top five reasons high school seniors did not use:

- They had no desire to use.
- Parents would object.
- Use is dangerous.
- Use is against their principles.
- They do not like the effects.

As we think about the messages we wish to send to the athletes who participate on our teams, it is helpful to consider the reasons why young people choose not to use. We can appeal to these motivations when we talk to young people about tobacco, alcohol, and other drugs.

Benefits of Choosing Not to Use

In our experience, focusing on these reasons and on other benefits for not using tobacco, alcohol, and other drugs is a more helpful approach than concentrating on the negative aspects of using. The following, adapted from Svendsen and Griffin (1990), are some of the benefits for choosing not to use.

Performance Will Not Be Hampered

When free of the influence of tobacco, alcohol, and other drugs, young people can perform a variety of tasks with full judgment and maximum physical skills, such as:

- Academics
- Athletics
- Music or dramatic arts
- Making decisions in everyday life situations
- Driving any kind of vehicle
- Operating equipment and tools

Tobacco, alcohol, and other drug use can diminish motivation, impair judgment, and directly reduce physical and intellectual performance in many areas.

The Risks of Experiencing Drug-Related Problems Are Reduced

A young adult who chooses not to use tobacco, alcohol, or other drugs will eliminate or reduce the risks of many of the following:

- Legal problems of underage use of tobacco, alcohol, or illicit drugs
- Dependency or addiction
- Involvement in an alcohol- or other drug-related traffic crash
- Involvement in an alcohol- or other drug-related swimming or boating accident
- Problems resulting from alcohol- or other drug-impaired sexual decisions

Life Skills Can Develop Completely

The adolescent who chooses to abstain from the use of tobacco, alcohol, and other drugs gains the best opportunity to develop skills in

- stress management,
- conflict resolution,
- problem solving, and
- goal setting.

Tobacco, alcohol, and other drug use can mistakenly mask problems and interfere with the development of these important life skills.

Physical, Emotional, Social, and Spiritual Development Can Occur Normally and Naturally

A young person's development of independence, self-responsibility, and meaning in life is best achieved without the interference of tobacco, alcohol, and other drugs. Examples include the following:

- Normal physiological and hormonal growth and development
- Appropriate moral and spiritual development
- Ability to solve life's daily problems and cope with stresses
- Ability to interact and get along with others

Tobacco, alcohol, and other drug use can disrupt healthy development and actually interfere with maturation.

Relationships Can Develop Honestly and Be Based on Mutual Interests

Young people who meet and talk together when sober and straight do not have to be concerned about the effect alcohol or other drugs might have on what they say or what is said to them. In fact, they will have the capacity to be open and honest. Positive results include the following:

- Morale of teams or groups will be enhanced.
- Sexual health problems, such as unplanned pregnancy, sexually transmitted diseases including AIDS, and acquaintance rape, will be reduced.
- People are less likely to say or do things to others they will later regret.
- Family standards and relationships will be strengthened.
- There will be no need to lie to others or to be secretive about drug use.

While none of these benefits alone are likely to persuade young people to choose not to use tobacco, alcohol, or other drugs, together they can allow you to share information that goes beyond the fact that drinking alcohol or using tobacco and other drugs is illegal for young people. Indeed, these reasons form the basis for why we have laws, rules, and athletic codes of conduct. These benefits can be communicated to young people one at a time by coaches, parents, teachers, relatives, clergy, employers, and any other adult in the community. Collectively, the same message by many messengers can have a powerful, positive influence on the choices young people make.

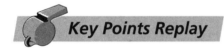 **Key Points Replay**

- Athletes probably are motivated to use tobacco, alcohol, and other drugs in the same way as other young people and may face additional pressures. Sports may put some young people in situations that increase their risk of using tobacco, alcohol, and other drugs.

- Many of the same reasons for choosing not to use are given by both college and high school athletes.

- Rules and laws are rarely given as the primary reason that young people do not use tobacco, alcohol, or other drugs.

- We can be most effective in our prevention efforts if we understand both the motivations that may cause some athletes to use and the reasons many choose not to use. By keeping these motivations and reasons in mind, we can help to reduce the impact of the motivations to use and promote the benefits of choosing not to use.

- Emphasizing the benefits of choosing not to use is probably a more acceptable approach to young people than giving them a long list of risks and hazards.

Part

II

Taking Action

Part I of *Coaches Guide to Drugs and Sport* presented athletics as a platform for reaching athletes and their parents with positive prevention messages. Part II puts this information to work for you by concentrating on five specific actions you can take to help prevent your athletes from using tobacco, alcohol, and other drugs.

These five strategies have been selected out of many possible actions that can be taken. We believe these strategies fit well within your legitimate role as a coach. They do not require extensive time, training, or expertise beyond what is already required for your coaching position.

As you read the next five chapters, you will learn how to set positive examples regarding the use and nonuse of tobacco, alcohol, and other drugs. You will examine the rules and codes that govern your team and assess how well these policies are working to deter young people from using. You will identify opportunities that arise during the season to talk about tobacco, alcohol, and other drugs with young athletes and their parents. You will explore actions that parents and athletes can take to prevent problems and ways to respond to athletes when you become concerned about them.

Chapter

3

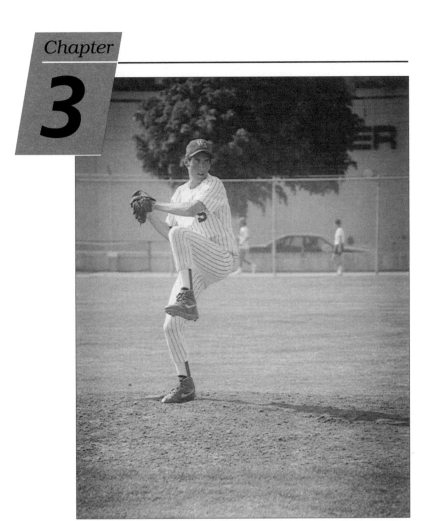

Setting a Positive Example

Chapter Warm-Up

Chapter 3 will help you set positive examples regarding the use and nonuse of tobacco, alcohol, and other drugs. You will examine how your own attitudes and behavior set an example for young people and be able to talk to your colleagues about the appropriate use or nonuse of tobacco, alcohol, and other drugs.

The Importance of Being Clear and Consistent

The overriding goal of *Coaches Guide to Drugs and Sport* is to work through athletics to send clear and consistent messages about tobacco, alcohol, and other drugs. The research is clear on this subject: If we expect young people to behave in a particular way, they need to obtain clear and consistent messages about the behavior we expect. Unfortunately, in our culture young people receive mixed messages about a number of behavioral issues, including sexuality, nutrition, violence, tobacco, alcohol, and other drugs. They receive these mixed messages in two distinct ways.

Different Sources Give Different Messages

Young people may get conflicting messages from peers, family, community, their culture, and the media. For instance, a young athlete may get an entirely different message about alcohol from watching the Super Bowl than from listening to the school's health teacher.

Receiving the same message from many messengers will have the most powerful impact on young people's behavior. Therefore, we need to provide ways that young people can receive positive messages about nonuse from a variety of credible sources in our communities. As a coach, you are an important source of information about tobacco, alcohol, and other drugs. Working in cooperation with parents, other school staff, and your athletes, you can increase the chances that young people will hear the same nonuse message many times from different people.

One Source Gives Conflicting Messages

Young people may also get a conflicting message from the same source. For instance, consider the mixed message given by a coach who says, "Tobacco use can impair your performance. Your endurance will dramatically decrease if you choose to smoke. Don't do it. And, by the way, don't let me catch you drinking." The message is mixed: Tobacco use is bad, but drinking alcohol is only bad if you're caught. Or consider the coach who tells young people that they do not have to drink to have a good time but celebrates every victory or drowns every defeat at the local bar. Young people discount our words if our actions are not consistent with those words. This section of *Coaches Guide to Drugs and Sport* will help you make sure your actions are consistent with the nonuse message you send to your athletes.

Setting Standards Through Example

Like it or not, many athletes, parents, and fans put coaches on a pedestal, expecting you to be exemplary in every aspect of your life. Fairly or unfairly, they look to you as a role model for the young people you coach. The drugs that are legal for adults, particularly alcohol and tobacco, seem to cause the most concern for coaches: Most coaches are over the legal age to use tobacco and alcohol and most of the young people they coach are not. Many coaches use alcohol, and most of those do so in a manner that does not cause problems for themselves or others around them. Should these coaches quit using alcohol to set a better example for the athletes they coach? If coaches use tobacco and alcohol, can they do so without sending a mixed message?

Ways to Set a Good Example

There are two ways that you can be a positive role model regarding tobacco, alcohol, and other drug use. You can either choose to abstain or decide to use those substances moderately, appropriately, and legally.

Choose Not to Use

Many adults do abstain from using tobacco, alcohol, or other drugs for a variety of reasons. Nearly one third of the adults in America choose to abstain from the use of alcohol (Figure 3.1). Over two thirds of American adults do not use tobacco products, and nearly 90% abstain from the use of any illicit drugs (U.S. Department of Health and Human Services, 1993). The assumption that "everyone drinks" or uses is simply not true. Abstaining from using tobacco, alcohol, and other drugs is one perfectly good way to be a positive role model for young people. Every person's choice to abstain—for whatever reason—should be protected and affirmed.

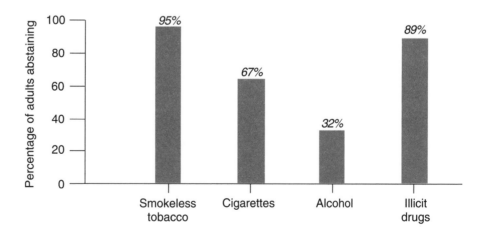

Figure 3.1   Adults who abstain from tobacco, alcohol, and other drug use.

Note. This data identifies those who have not used within the past year as "abstainers." It is compiled from information on 21,578 people over the age of 18. Although 18-20 year olds are not legally considered adults, this category is not divided from the total sample.

Compiled from U.S. Department of Health and Human Services (1993).

Use Appropriately, Moderately, and Legally

Choosing to use tobacco, alcohol, and other drugs appropriately, moderately, and legally is another way to be a good role model for young people. However, many factors, such as personal experience, use by family and peers, religious values or personal beliefs, community and cultural norms, and laws or rules shape what different people consider to be appropriate and moderate. Because of this, it is often difficult to draw the line between use and misuse of tobacco, alcohol, and other drugs. In order to send clear and consistent messages to young people, adults must work to clarify this line. We must be able to give two messages to young people: As a young person, you should not use tobacco, alcohol, or other drugs. As an adult, if you decide to use, do so appropriately, moderately, and legally.

American culture often has divided alcohol use into two categories: wet, dry; good, bad; right, wrong. Although these distinctions may be helpful to support the actions of those who choose not to use, they provide no guidance to those who wish to use moderately and appropriately. This view implies that what one third of the adult population (the nonusers) is doing is right and that the actions of two thirds are wrong. In fact, the majority of adults who use alcohol do so legally, appropriately, and moderately. Approximately 6% to 10% of the adult population is alcohol dependent and about 20% experiences other problems with their use. It appears that approximately 40% of the adult population uses alcohol with no serious negative consequences. If our goal in prevention is to prevent problems associated with tobacco, alcohol, and other drugs, then the likely allies in this effort are nonusers and those who choose to use appropriately, moderately, and legally—approximately 70% of the adults in our country (Figure 3.2).

Where Do You Draw the Line?

30%   Nonuse

--- Here?

40%   Use appropriately

--- Or here?

20%   Misuse (Use + Problems)

10%   Addiction (Use + Problems + Loss of Control)

Figure 3.2   Categories of adult use and nonuse of alcohol.

Reprinted from Harding, Ringhofer & Associates, Inc., 1994.

Setting Personal Guidelines

The following are some suggested guidelines for helping you set positive standards for the use and nonuse of tobacco, alcohol, and

A standard is something that is established by custom, general consent, or authority as a model or example to follow.

other drugs. We offer these guidelines in order to clarify the concepts of legal, appropriate, and moderate use and to help you avoid risky situations. These guidelines are adapted from the TARGET Leadership Training Manual (Harding, Ringhofer & Associates, Inc., 1994).

"Legal" is relatively easy to define, even though laws may change. Age limits make some drugs, including alcohol and tobacco, illegal for minors. Other drugs are illegal for everyone, regardless of age. When use is legal, then criteria for "moderate" and "appropriate" need to be applied. These are more difficult to determine. Figure 3.3 shows each term's parameters.

Appropriate = Time and Place

Moderate = Amount and Frequency

Figure 3.3   Appropriate and moderate parameters.

1. There are circumstances when nonuse is the only appropriate choice. You should abstain from alcohol if you are

   - under age 21,
   - chemically dependent,
   - pregnant or nursing,
   - using medications that warn against alcohol use,
   - driving motorized vehicles,
   - operating dangerous equipment,
   - at work or school, or
   - performing in fine arts or physical activities.

   You should avoid tobacco use (including smokeless tobacco) and discourage others—regardless of age—from using tobacco products. Tobacco use has specific health and social risks. Even though tobacco is legal for adults and some people claim to use it moderately and appropriately, very few escape being caught by the highly addictive substance—nicotine—which is present in all tobacco products. Each year in the United States more people die from tobacco-related causes than from the effects of all other drugs combined.

   You should also avoid any use of illicit drugs and discourage others from using these drugs. In general, these drugs are illegal because of the serious risks associated with their use. Because they are illegal, the dosage and purity of illicit drugs is unpredictable, which increases health and social risks. Both possession and use also have significant legal and ethical risks.

2. There are times when the use of alcohol or other drugs may be appropriate.

   • When your personal values or religious beliefs accept the use of alcohol or other drugs.

   • When use is legal.

   • When use is a minor part of other activities (such as a beverage at mealtimes).

   • When it is part of religious ceremonies or cultural traditions.

   • When your participation in current or upcoming events (such as driving, studying, working, supervising young people, or participation in physical activities) will not be impaired by use.

   • When drugs are prescribed by a physician or used as directed on an over-the-counter package. Medications should be disposed of after the expiration date and should never be shared or exchanged with others.

   • When use will not affect others in a negative way.

3. If you choose to use, do so moderately to avoid intoxication and other negative effects.

   Intoxication is unhealthy and risky. Avoid intoxication yourself, and discourage others from becoming intoxicated.

   If you choose to drink or to serve alcohol to others, take into consideration the factors that influence the effects of alcohol. These factors include the following:

   • Alcohol content

   • Number of drinks and time between drinks

   • Weight, age, and gender of the individual

   • Situational factors, such as food eaten, fatigue, or emotional state

   As a general rule of thumb, you can avoid intoxication by consuming no more than 12 ounces of regular beer, 5 ounces of wine, or 1.5 ounces of 80-proof distilled spirits per hour. Moderate drinking guidelines also limit the number of alcoholic drinks per day. As shown in Figure 3.4, the American Dietary Guidelines (U.S. Department of Agriculture and U.S. Department of Health and Human Services, 1991) suggest no more than one drink per day for women, and no more than two drinks per day for men. The Michigan Office of Substance Abuse Prevention suggests no more than three drinks per day, and discourages daily drinking. Their Zero, One, Three campaign also suggests times when people should abstain from any alcohol use (Figure 3.5).

4. Regardless of whether or not we choose to use, others' use may affect us. There are ways to reduce personal risk from those who use inappropriately.

   • Impaired drivers—Always wear your seat belts. Avoid riding with an impaired driver. Be cautious of driving at bar closing times.

What is moderate drinking?

Women

No more than 1 drink a day

Men

No more than 2 drinks a day

What is one drink?

1.5 ounces of distilled spirits (80 proof)

5 ounces of wine

12 ounces of regular beer

Figure 3.4   U.S. guidelines.

Reprinted from U.S. Department of Agriculture and U.S. Department of Health and Human Services (1991).

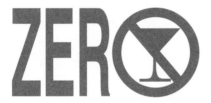

Zero = Zero alcohol. Especially if you are under 21, driving, chemically dependent, or pregnant.

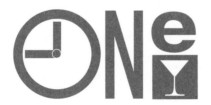

One = One drink per hour sets the pace for moderate drinking.

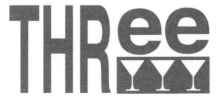

Three = No more than three drinks in one day, and never drink alcohol daily.

Figure 3.5   Zero, One, Three guidelines.

Adapted from material developed by Enjoy Michigan Safely Coalition.

- High-risk sexual situations—Avoid solo situations with someone who is intoxicated. Plan ahead to circumvent a high-risk situation.
- Secondary smoke—Ask smokers to respect your right to a smoke-free environment. Request nonsmoking areas in restaurants and hotels.
- Misuse by friends and family members—Seek help for yourself from a professional or through Al-Anon, a support group for those who are affected by others' use of tobacco, alcohol, and other drugs.

5. We can help others make healthy choices about tobacco, alcohol and other drugs.

- Do not allow tobacco, alcohol, and other drugs to become the primary focus of events. It is not necessary to celebrate special occasions by using any drug, including alcohol, nor is it necessary to serve alcohol at mealtimes or during other family or social events.
- If you choose to serve alcohol, minimize the health and safety risks for your guests. "Non-Alcoholic Party Drinks," available from the Minnesota Prevention Resource Center, gives hosting tips and recipes for non-alcoholic drinks (Minnesota Prevention Resource Center, 1985).
- Prevent others from driving while intoxicated by offering them a ride, calling a cab, taking their keys, or calling a police officer.
- If you choose to use, model standards for appropriate and moderate use.
- Respect and affirm the rights of others to choose not to use or to use moderately and appropriately. No one should be pressured to drink or to use or be made to feel uneasy because of their personal choice. No one needs to justify the choice. However, it can be helpful under certain circumstances to share reasons for choosing not to use alcohol or other drugs.
- Talk to others when you are concerned about their use of tobacco, alcohol, or other drugs.
- Use teachable moments to discuss tobacco, alcohol, or other drug use or nonuse. Chapter 5 provides information about using teachable moments with athletes.

It requires maturity and responsibility to establish guidelines and limits before beginning to use. This is a primary reason for having an age limit on the use of certain substances, like alcohol. If we expect an age limit to make any sense to young people under the age limit, those of legal age should model positive ways to use and not use. Table 3.1 gives some suggestions for "when is when." These suggestions may be helpful for reinforcing or redefining personal guidelines and for establishing healthy community standards.

Table 3.1 When is When? A Guide To Alcohol Use and Nonuse		
Say "No"	**Say "Maybe"**	**Know "When Is When"**
There are times when "no" is the only appropriate choice:	*There are times when use of alcohol "may be" appropriate:*	*If we choose to use alcohol, then we must use moderately.*
1. When use is illegal, including underage drinking 2. When the person is recovering from dependency or addiction 3. When a woman is pregnant or nursing 4. When medications warn against alcohol use 5. When driving motorized vehicles or operating dangerous equipment 6. While at work or at school 7. When performing in fine arts or physical activities	1. When personal values or religious beliefs accept the use of alcohol 2. When use is legal 3. When use is a minor part of other activities (such as a beverage at mealtimes) 4. When use is part of a religious ceremony or cultural tradition 5. When participation in upcoming events will not be impaired by use 6. When use will not affect others in a negative way	1. Intoxication is unhealthy, risky, and should be avoided and discouraged 2. One drink per hour is all a person's body can detoxify. One drink = 5 oz of wine, one 12-oz bottle of beer, or 1.5 oz of 80-proof liquor. 3. One guideline for alcohol use suggests that no more than three drinks per day should be consumed. The American Dietary Council recommends one drink per day for women and two for men. 4. Daily drinking should be avoided. 5. Do not drink on an empty stomach; food slows the rate of absorption. 6. Reduce or eliminate alcohol use during times of depression, anger, or fatigue.

Reprinted from Ringhofer & Harding, 1993.

By following such guidelines we will become better able to explain our choices in a way which is rational and helpful to young people. If we choose to use appropriately, moderately, and legally, we will be able to say more than "It's legal for me and illegal for you." Our actions and our words will be more consistent for young people.

Coming to Consensus With Your Colleagues

In addition to establishing personal guidelines, you can discuss these guidelines with your colleagues. If you and your colleagues can agree to certain practices as a group, this can send a more consistent message to others, including your athletes. Some examples of standards that you might agree to are the following:

- If a meeting for coaches is held in place where alcohol is served, we will conduct the business meeting before alcohol is consumed.

- All banquets and award functions where youth are present will take place in an area that is free of all drugs, particularly alcohol and nicotine.

- We will not use alcohol, tobacco, or other drugs when we are chaperoning (or otherwise responsible for) athletes, including overnight trips.

- We will not use illegal drugs.

- If we do choose to use alcohol, we will do so moderately and appropriately, following guidelines such as those suggested above.

Any guidelines on which you and your colleagues can agree will help your coaching staff send a more consistent message about tobacco, alcohol, and other drugs. We suggest that you work on these agreements without those in positions of authority present. For a group of coaches, your athletic director would not attend. If someone in position of authority is present, the focus of the discussion usually turns to what the authority can expect and enforce. Often a group of colleagues may come to agreements that go beyond contracts, rules, or expectations of authorities.

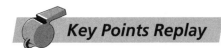

Key Points Replay

- You are a role model for your athletes. What you say and do can influence their decisions about tobacco, alcohol, and other drugs.

- You can be a good role model in two ways: by choosing not to use tobacco, alcohol, or other drugs or by using them appropriately, moderately, and legally.

- There are times, however, when abstinence is the only appropriate choice.

- Standards often are not clear in our communities about what constitutes appropriate and moderate use of tobacco, alcohol, and other drugs. We often send mixed messages to young people.

- You can work with your colleagues to agree to standards that send a more consistent message about tobacco, alcohol, and other drugs.

4

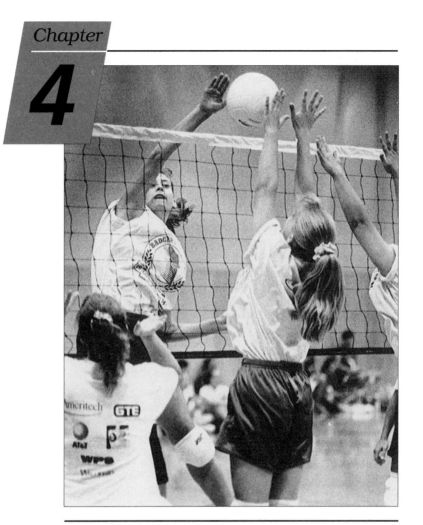

Establishing and Enforcing Rules

Chapter Warm-Up

Chapter 4 will help you establish and enforce rules for effective deterrence. You will explore some of the basic components of preventive codes of conduct and be able to give a rationale for rules and their consequences. You will feel more prepared to enforce rules fairly and consistently and be able to work with others to write or revise athletic policies, if necessary. You will gather ideas for expanding the methods you use to communicate rules to athletes and their parents.

The Purpose of Codes of Conduct

The purpose of codes of conduct and rules about tobacco, alcohol and other drugs is to help people make good decisions. A code of conduct that is well conceived, properly written, and thoroughly communicated does just that. It sets standards of behavior for everyone involved in athletics. These standards provide guidance for young people as they make choices about tobacco, alcohol, and other drugs and provide direction for important adults who support young athletes.

The purpose of a code of conduct is not to eliminate athletes who engage in inappropriate behavior. Yet, many athletic programs develop and enforce codes of conduct as if this were their intention. With severe penalties and no opportunity for education or help, they attempt to eliminate the "bad apples" from their teams. As we have seen in chapter 2, many of the athletes on our teams choose to use tobacco, alcohol, and other drugs, even during the season. It is not just the "bad kids" who use. All of our athletes can benefit from codes that set a standard of nonuse and provide corrective action when the standard is violated.

A code of conduct should encompass a wide range of behaviors that the school and community have deemed appropriate or inappropriate for student athletes. It is obviously wrong to bench an athlete for using tobacco, alcohol, or other drugs while a teammate who has been convicted of assault, theft, or vandalism is allowed to play. However, this chapter will limit its attention to rules as they apply to tobacco, alcohol, and other drugs.

As much as possible, the focus of rules should be on prevention. As its first course of action, rules should seek to deter athletes from using drugs and, secondarily, apply consequences when the rules are violated. Rules should also help identify young people who are experiencing problems with tobacco, alcohol, and other drugs and provide avenues for them to obtain help to resolve these problems.

Special Codes of Conduct for Athletes

Most schools have formal policies and procedures for handling student use of tobacco, alcohol, and other drugs, but most schoolwide policies only address on-campus use, possession, and sale of substances. This chapter will discuss athletic codes and policies which go beyond rules that apply to nonathletes.

In most cases, the courts have upheld the right of school cocurricular activities to have expectations for participants that exceed those of the general student body. Courts have based their rulings on the fact that cocurricular activities are a privilege, not a right, and that schools can therefore have higher expectations for these students. These expectations can extend to the off-campus activities of cocurricular participants. For example, courts have ruled that an athletic program may suspend an athlete for drinking alcohol at a weekend party if the athletic rules and procedures have been clearly communicated to the athlete prior to the incident.

Keys to Effective Rules

Research from the criminal justice system has shown that laws most effectively prevent problems when they are consistently enforced, when consequences for violations are perceived as fair, and when the process is prompt.

A good example of these principles in action is the reaction of our country to the change in marijuana laws. Prior to the mid-1970s, possession of even a small amount of marijuana was considered a felony. A young person who was caught in possession of marijuana was arrested, charged, and sentenced with a crime that would remain permanently on his or her record. As marijuana use began to be more widespread, people in many communities began to believe that the punishment did not fit this particular crime. Consequently, even police officers did not consistently enforce the law, and many young people perceived—rightfully so—that they would not get caught or be penalized if they possessed or used marijuana. When the charge was dropped to a misdemeanor, young people were required to pay a small fine and, often, to attend an educational session. More police officers were willing to enforce a law that would provide more reasonable consequences. Arrests increased. This approach, coupled with many other prevention efforts, led to a decline in current marijuana use from a high of 37.1% in 1978 to an all-time low of 11.9% in 1992 (Johnston, O'Malley, & Bachman, 1994).

Consequences Are Perceived as Fair

The perception of fair and reasonable consequences is the linchpin in this process, affecting both consistent and prompt enforcement. Many people believe that more severe penalties have a greater deterrent effect—if the penalty is harsh enough, no one will dare break the rule. Research on the relationship between penalties and crime reduction has not shown this to be true, nor does it appear to be true in athletics. Kicking an athlete off a team for tobacco, alcohol, or other drug use does not necessarily prevent use but may prevent enforcement of the rule. Coaches often perceive—correctly—that athletics keep some young people in school. Coaches may also realize that they are some of the most significant adults in some young people's lives. For some students, athletic scholarships ride on their performance. Therefore, coaches are reluctant to kick a young person off a team, knowing that an athlete is likely to quit school, lose a chance at a college education, or that they will be unable to remain a positive influence in that young person's life.

So what are fair and reasonable consequences? A tongue-in-cheek answer: What is fair and reasonable is whatever you are willing to apply to all athletes. Rules are sometimes made with the "bad" athlete in mind; he is the one you may not want to have on your team anyway. Instead, they should be created for all athletes, including your "best" players and those who may make mistakes.

Consequences must be survivable, and coaches—who have the ultimate good of the young person in mind—must believe that they are survivable.

There Is Consistent Enforcement

When coaches perceive that consequences for a rule infraction are fair and reasonable, they are more likely to consistently enforce the rule. When players perceive that the consequences are fair and reasonable, they are more likely to be honest. When parents perceive that the consequences are appropriate, they are more likely to support the coach. However, if coaches, parents, and players believe that the consequences are too stiff or unfair, they are likely to turn their heads the other way or find a way around the consequences. Many adolescents believe they are invincible. They often believe that consequences happen to other people and that they will not get caught. When young athletes perceive that coaches will enforce a rule and that there will actually be consequences for breaking the rule, the rule can have a deterrent effect.

Consistent enforcement must be upheld by you as an individual coach and by the entire coaching staff. You must examine how consistent you are among players, striving to make sure you enforce the rule and apply the consequences to all players equally. The coaching staff must look at consistency among teams to make sure that athletes are not getting by with infractions on one team while the same behavior is severely punished on another team.

As schools work to achieve consistency, many develop policies that govern participants in all cocurricular activities. This sends a more consistent message to young people and dispels any belief that we are either "fingering" or "favoring" athletes by our policies and programs.

The Process Is Prompt

Also, for a rule to deter behavior, the consequences for violating it must happen quickly. Adolescents, in particular, need immediacy. An investigation which drags on for weeks is less effective in either changing or preventing behavior. When coaches perceive that a rule and its consequences are fair, they will be more likely to step in quickly and take action. When parents and students perceive that the consequences for violating a rule are fair and reasonable, they are far more likely to simply accept the consequences. If they do not think the consequences are fair and just, they may fight the rule, even to the extent of taking the school to court.

What is prompt? The procedures should specify how long each of the various actions should take, keeping in mind that an adolescent's perception of prompt is much shorter than an adult's.

Two weeks or a month can seem like an eternity to an adolescent. Action should take place as soon as the behavior comes to the attention of the coach, with contact made with the student and parents (when appropriate) within 48 hours (or within 48 hours of the school's start, if the incident happens over the weekend). The school's due process should be followed. Decisions on the appropriate action should happen as soon as enough information has been gathered, with consequences beginning immediately after the decision has been made. In most cases, this should not take longer than one week.

A good example of these principles in action is the reaction one community had when it dropped its "death penalty" from its athletic code. In this school, the athletic code required athletes to be suspended from participating in all athletic activities for one season if they used even a small amount of tobacco, alcohol, or other drugs. It became common knowledge that most coaches would not enforce this policy, so people could only remember a few times that an athlete was actually suspended from a team. As a result of advice from parents, students, and coaches, the consequences of violating the rule on the first offense were changed to suspending athletes for two games and requiring them to practice with the team during their suspension. Just after the start of the fall season, rumors were rampant that drinking parties were taking place and that many athletes were participating in them. The hockey coach had a meeting with his prospective players and asked them to be honest about whether or not they had been attending the parties and whether or not they had been drinking alcohol. The next day, the community was shocked when 20 players "turned themselves in." They were consequently suspended from two weeks of play. Because some of them were also football players and, therefore, did not participate during their football games, the football coach was not pleased. That, however, is another story.

In this example, if the coach had been required to suspend his players for the season, would he have gone out of his way to meet with his athletes about this issue? Would 20 of his players have stepped forward? If he had then suspended all of these athletes, how would the parents have reacted? How would the football coach have responded if he had lost part of his team for the entire season? Would the hockey coach have been willing to take the flack from parents, other coaches, and his team? Or would it have been easier to simply ignore the rumor because he did not have proof?

Working With Others to Create or Revise an Athletic Code of Conduct

Codes of conduct for athletes may be written and administered from several different levels. The following information is adapted from the TARGET Leadership Training Manual (Harding, Ringhofer & Associates, Inc., 1994).

Statewide Rules or Codes of Conduct

If you coach in one of a handful of states, your team will be expected to uphold statewide rules that govern the use of tobacco, alcohol, and other drugs by athletes or participants in other cocurricular activities. These rules are developed by the state athletic or activity association and provide a minimum standard for violation of policies regarding the use of tobacco, alcohol, and other drugs. Although it is generally discouraged, school districts may adopt a policy that has more severe penalties than the statewide rule. Policies written at a statewide level tend to minimize unfair competition among schools, because schools are required to apply the policy uniformly to all athletes. This also tends to make the messages that athletes get about tobacco, alcohol, and other drugs more consistent. If you coach in one of these states, your school should still have a formal policy that references the rule and specifies the exact procedures to follow if a violation of the policy occurs. However, most of the development and administration of this policy will be on the shoulders of the athletic or activity administrator. You should, however, be proactive in voicing your opinion about how your school's rules are written and communicated to your athletes and their parents.

Districtwide Rules Governing Athletics

In some states, schools have the liberty of writing and adopting their own policies on a school-by-school basis. In a few cases, your state athletic or activity association will mandate that your school have a policy in place, or they will recommend a policy. When policies are written at the school-district level, the responsibility for developing or implementing the policy usually falls on the shoulders of the athletic director or another administrator. As policies are written and implemented, you should advocate that coaches from all teams have a voice in creating the policy, along with team members and their parents. You still need to communicate the rule, its rationale, and its importance to your players and their parents.

Team-By-Team Codes of Conduct

In some cases, athletic codes are written and administered team-by-team, coach-by-coach. This option lends itself to miscommunication and misunderstanding because many students are involved in more than one sport or more than one activity. Athletes may receive mixed messages from different coaches about what is appropriate or inappropriate behavior concerning tobacco, alcohol, and other drug use. On the other hand, if rules are developed by each team, the coach may have more ownership in enforcing them. If you are in this situation, then you will most likely be directly responsible for writing and communicating rules to your athletes and their parents. The following action steps will be yours to take. These steps can also be used if you are part of a group working on codes of conduct for all teams or all school activities in a school district.

Step One: Establish a Planning Group

It may be much more expedient for you to simply write a policy and distribute it to athletes and their parents than to struggle through the process of developing a policy by consensus. However, what you gain in expediency in the beginning, you will most likely lose in the end through lack of support for the policy. A planning group should consist of whomever is affected by it: school board representatives, administrators (including your athletic administrator), teachers, coaches, parents, athletes, your school's student assistance coordinator, other counseling staff members and/or prevention specialists, law enforcement officials, assessment and treatment agencies, and other community representatives.

Step Two: Learn About Prevention

This planning group needs to have an opportunity to learn about effective codes and policies because group members will often take the position that tougher is better. Students are especially prone to adopting a "kick-them-off-the-team" approach until it comes time to apply this consequence to their friends or themselves. You may want to suggest that members of the planning group read the parts of this chapter that apply to fair, consistent, and prompt enforcement.

Step Three: Review Existing Policies and Programs

This group must also take the time to become familiar with policies and programs that already exist within the school and community in order to craft a code that is consistent with the community's philosophy and available resources. State laws about tobacco, alcohol, and other drugs; state association policies and guidelines; school disciplinary policies (including right to due process); and student-assistance program policies are especially relevant. The athletic code or policy should dovetail nicely with these policies.

Step Four: Write and Disseminate Your First Draft

Once the large group has verbally given input for the development of the policy, a small team should write the rule. It should address the following areas:

- The philosophy of the planning group for developing the rule
- The reason the rule is being written
- The types of drugs that are prohibited, the actions that are prohibited, and the time period the rule will be in effect
- The consequences of a violation
- Other prevention strategies that are associated with athletics

Once the first draft is written, it should be given back to the larger team, which is responsible for taking it back to its constituent groups.

For instance, student-athlete representatives may take the rule back to their teams for reaction. Parent representatives may take the rule to the booster club. Coaches may take the rule back to a staff meeting. At this point, legal counsel should also be sought to review the policy.

Step Five: Revise and Submit the Final Code

Once the rule has been disseminated and various groups have had a chance to review and comment, the planning group will meet once again to discuss the responses they received. The writing team will then take the responses and revise the rule until it meets the satisfaction of the planning group, after which time it will be submitted to whomever must give final approval. In the case of an individual coach, the final authority may be the athletic director. In other cases, the school board must have final approval.

Step Six: Communicate the Policy and Procedures

If the previous steps have been followed, then communication is easier. The awareness of the athletic policy should be widespread because most people will have seen one of the earlier versions of the policy. Unveiling the final code should be a well-publicized event because it will be a teachable moment for everyone involved. The following information presents many options for repeatedly communicating rules and their consequences throughout the season.

Communicating Rules to Athletes and Their Parents

Rules and their consequences must be communicated clearly and simply to athletes and parents prior to and during each season. Athletes and their parents need to know what the coaches expect and what will happen if those expectations are not met.

No matter what methods are used to communicate rules, it is important for athletes and their parents to know the reasons for having rules that prohibit the use of tobacco, alcohol, and other drugs. The rationale for a given rule helps young people know that a rule is not simply something made up by adults to spoil their fun; rules are made with concern for their health and safety. Tobacco products and alcoholic beverages are illegal for adolescents primarily because they pose greater risks to the health and safety of young people than adults. There is also evidence that the younger a person starts to use, the more likely that person will experience more severe problems later with use. Other drugs, such as performance-altering drugs (anabolic androgenic steroids), may be prohibited in order to prevent athletes from getting an unfair advantage over others. The following is one example of how the rationale for a rule was written.

Rationale

"This school district recognizes that the use of tobacco, alcohol, and other drugs interferes with the physical, intellectual, social, and emotional development of our community's young people. Reflecting the prevention philosophy of both our athletic program and our school system, this policy's intent is to send a clear and consistent message to all athletes, coaches, parents, and program administrators regarding tobacco, alcohol, and other drugs. The adolescent use of tobacco, alcohol, and other drugs is illegal and presents a significant threat to an athlete's health and safety and to the orderly conduct of athletic programs. The additional safety factors associated with active, competitive participation give the athletic community an added responsibility to provide the safest and healthiest environment for all concerned." (Adapted from City of Warwick Athletic Policy, Warwick, RI, 1992.)

Taking the time to explain the reasons you think rules are important can be one way you can express your concern for your athletes. Your opinion that young people should not use tobacco, alcohol, and other drugs is probably more important to young athletes and their parents than the rule itself. Yet rules provide an opportunity for you to show your concern and state your opinion.

There are many ways to communicate rules both prior to and during the season. Here are a few suggestions:

Written Methods

Most schools routinely publish their policies in student handbooks with the expectation that students and parents will read, understand, and agree to the contents. Some athletic programs also publish athletic handbooks and include their codes of conduct. Rules may also be published in a school newsletter or community newspaper. The problem with these methods of communicating rules and policies is that often parents and students do not take the time to read and consider these rules on an annual basis. Signed statements are one way of boosting the chance the rules will be read. These statements simply acknowledge that the parents and athletes have received, read, and understood the policy. Here is an example:

Acknowledgment

"I have read, understand, and acknowledge receiving the *1994-1995 Athletic Eligibility Information*, which contains a summary of the eligibility rules of the Minnesota State High School League. These rules prohibit the use of tobacco, alcohol, and other drugs during the year by any participant in Minnesota athletic programs" (Minnesota State High School League, 1994).

When you say nothing, what do athletes hear? "The coach just doesn't care about anything except how well I can play," or "The coach didn't say anything about it, so we thought it was OK."

Written contracts may go further and ask parents and athletes to abide by the conditions set forth in the code of conduct. Athletes agree that they will not use tobacco, alcohol, and other drugs and that they will abide by the consequences if they choose to violate the code. Signing this contract is required in order to participate. Parents agree to uphold the contract. They differ from voluntary pledges, discussed in chapter 6, which are generally not a condition of team membership. Here is an example:

Participant Contract

"I, _____ , have chosen to participate in basketball at North High School. I commit myself to continuously working toward the goal of top physical fitness. To do anything which would harm my body would not be in my best interest or the best interest of my team and school. I agree to remain free from tobacco, alcohol, and other drugs during my sports season. I fully understand this pledge extends to seven days per week. If I have a problem or need help fulfilling this contract, I understand that the coaches, the substance-abuse coordinator, and school counselors will be available to help me. I have read and understand the athletic policies and the consequences for violations of these policies. I pledge to keep all rules and policies and to help all of my teammates abide by the same athletic rules and policies.

"As the parent/guardian of _____ , I understand and support this contract and pledge that my son/daughter has signed. Optimum health is the goal of our athletic program, and I support the school system in its efforts to attain this goal" (National Federation TARGET Program, 1993b).

Visual Reminders

Knowing that people often forget what they have read once, some coaches print posters of the code of conduct and post them in the locker room and gymnasium. This can serve as a constant reminder of the code for both participants and fans. When athletes are involved in setting annual goals for their team, some coaches print wallet cards that may also include a reminder of the codes of conduct.

Formal Meetings

Preseason meetings are perhaps the best way to communicate rules and their rationale to students and their parents. Preseason meetings can also be an opportunity to distribute and collect signed contracts from athletes and their parents. Other team meetings, held throughout the year, can be used to discuss these codes of conduct. Chapter 5 provides detailed information on conducting preseason meetings.

Informal Discussions

Informal opportunities that come up throughout the year can be used to communicate and reinforce your rules to your players. When you hear rumors about an upcoming party, this can be a time to talk to athletes about your concern for them and your expectation that they not use. When a rule infraction takes place, this can be a time to discuss the rule and to remind athletes that their commitment to the team includes choosing not to use tobacco, alcohol, and other drugs. Using these teachable moments is further discussed in chapter 5.

Special Considerations

The following information provides guidance on special issues that arise as you develop or revise rules about tobacco, alcohol, and other drugs.

Progressive Steps

Most policies include progressive consequences for subsequent violations. This progression should also include increasingly intensive efforts to determine if the student has a problem with tobacco, alcohol, or other drugs and to provide assistance to resolve such problems (see "Student Assistance Program Referral," pp. 48-49).

Progressive Steps

"First Violation: After confirmation of the first violation, the student shall lose eligibility for the next two (2) consecutive interscholastic contests or two (2) weeks of a season in which the student is a participant, whichever is greater.

"Second Violation: After confirmation of the second violation, the student shall lose eligibility for the next six (6) consecutive interscholastic contests in which the student is a participant.

"Third and Subsequent Violations: After confirmation of the third or subsequent violations, the student shall lose eligibility for the next twelve (12) consecutive interscholastic contests in which the student is a participant" (Minnesota State High School League, 1994).

Effective Time Period

How long is your rule in effect? Do you expect—through your rule—that a student athlete will not use tobacco, alcohol, and other drugs 365 days a year? For the full school year? Or for just the season of play (from the initial practice through the final contest, including tournaments)?

Effective Time Period

"This policy applies to the entire school year and any portion of an activity season which occurs prior to the start of the school year or after the close of the school year" (Minnesota State High School League, 1991).

Accumulation of Penalties

Will the penalties carry over from year to year? For instance, if a junior basketball player violates the same policy which that player violated as a freshman, does this constitute a second violation? Must the violation occur in the same year?

Penalty Accumulation

"Penalties shall be accumulative beginning with the student's first participation in a League activity and continuing through the student's high school career" (Minnesota State High School League, 1994).

Helping Clauses and Connection to the Student Assistance Program

A referral to a student assistance program should be made on every violation so that someone outside of the athletic program can determine if there is a pattern of tobacco, alcohol, or other drug use which may require further intervention, including treatment for chemical dependency (see Part III for more information on student assistance programs). The actions taken by the student assistance team and the athletic program may differ for each violation. Here are some examples:

Student Assistance Program Referral

"First Violation: The athlete will be directed to the school-based Student Assistance Program for assessment and possible referral. Prior to returning to competition, a form must be signed and presented to the athletic department indicating that progress is under way" (City of Warwick, RI).

"Second Violation: It is recommended that, prior to being re-admitted to activities, the student shall show evidence in writing that he/she has sought or has received counseling from a community agency or professional individual, such as a school counselor, drug counselor, medical doctor, psychiatrist, or psychologist. It is recommended that, when appropriate, the school refer a student to a community agency or a professional individual outside the school for assessment of potential chemical abuse or misuse" (Minnesota State High School League, 1990).

In the interest of providing help for troubled young people, including those who are chemically dependent, athletic participation is sometimes used as a hammer to force athletes into treatment. Although this approach can indeed be effective, it has financial and legal risks. In the athletic policy or student assistance policy, it should be made clear that assessment or treatment outside of the school setting is at the athlete's and the parents' discretion and, therefore, their expense. Federal and state laws governing data privacy, confidentiality, due process, and a student's right to an education must be upheld. Seek legal guidance as you develop both athletic and student assistance policies.

Reduced Penalties in Exchange for Participation in Counseling

For at least the first violation, for which penalties are usually relatively short, there should be no reduction of consequences for entering or participating in a counseling or treatment program. Decreasing consequences for students who are chemically dependent could be perceived as unfair. A student athlete who had his first drink at a party could end up being suspended while an athlete who drinks to intoxication every weekend could play as a result of an assessment which indicated that she needed counseling or treatment.

Counseling and Penalties

"First Violation: No exception is permitted for a student who becomes a participant in a treatment program.

If, after the second or subsequent violation, the student on his/her own accord becomes a participant in an approved chemical dependency program or treatment program, the student may be certified for reinstatement in MIAA activities after a minimum period of six (6) weeks. Such certification must be issued by the director or a counselor of a chemical dependency treatment center" (Massachusetts Interscholastic Athletic Association, 1993).

Practicing

Athletes should continue to practice with their team for a variety of reasons. Foremost is a need to protect the health and safety of the student athlete. It would not be appropriate to bar an athlete from practice and then return that athlete to play following the suspension without proper conditioning. Also, it is important for the athlete to stay in contact with you and the teammates as essential sources of support. If the athlete feels embarrassed about the incident, it may actually be more difficult for that athlete to participate in practice than to simply "disappear" for the length of the penalty. If athletes are in inpatient treatment, or otherwise removed from your supervision for an extended period of time, you will need to make certain that the athlete is in acceptable physical condition before returning to play.

Practice Participation

"The athlete will remain at practice for rehabilitation purposes, safety, and health reasons. If he/she plans to continue participating at the end of the suspension, continued practice/participation will make the individual ready to play at the conclusion of the suspension" (City of Warwick, RI).

Dishonesty

Most rule violations come to the attention of coaches through rumors or reports by another student, parent, or community member. Less frequently will you actually observe a student athlete consuming tobacco, alcohol, or other drugs. Therefore, enforcement of these policies and codes may rest on the honesty of the players when they are confronted about their use. Some schools build into their policy a dishonesty clause which allows them to increase penalties if a student is confronted about use, denies using, and is later found to have been dishonest.

Dishonesty

"A student shall be disqualified from all interscholastic athletics for nine (9) additional weeks beyond the student's original period of ineligibility when the student denies violation of the rule, is allowed to participate, and then is subsequently found guilty of the violation" (Minnesota State High School League, 1994).

Guilt by Association

If an athlete attends a party where tobacco, alcohol, and other drugs are consumed, is that athlete in violation of the policy? This policy may be easier to enforce; no one must prove that a young person was actually consuming alcohol or using other drugs. However, the essential fairness of this policy is often questioned by students and parents. Some nonusing athletes have also questioned the policy's wisdom, believing that they can positively influence other athletes if they can attend parties where tobacco, alcohol, or other drugs are present.

Self-Referral

Some policies allow consequences to be applied differently—or not at all—if a student athlete voluntarily comes forward to you, your athletic director, or some other designated staff member. Under some policies, if an athlete tells you of a drinking or drug problem, needs help, and no specific incidents of policy violations were disclosed, this athlete may be referred to counseling and not be subject to any penalties. Some policies simply allow for a one-time self-referral without consequences, whether or not a specific incident is disclosed. However, you must be careful to determine if this "admittance of a problem" is simply a Monday-morning attempt to dodge the consequences of drinking alcohol at a weekend party.

Investigating Rule Violations

Schools are not courts of law. They are, therefore, held to a much less stringent need to actually prove that a violation has occurred. You do not have to actually catch an athlete in the act of consuming tobacco, alcohol, or other drugs. Here are the general steps to follow when you hear of a possible violation:

- Do not ignore it. Even if the information comes to you as a rumor, you can still investigate. If someone else reports the incident to you, you must investigate. And, if an athlete comes to you and admits to violating the policy, you need to take action. Ignoring any of these three circumstances will give the impression that you are not serious about preventing tobacco, alcohol, or other drug use.

- If you are investigating a rumor, check it out with other sources until you are reasonably sure that the information is accurate. Then talk to the athlete or athletes who are involved, giving them a chance to be honest with you. The "Sharing Concern Process" in chapter 7 gives a structure for talking to an athlete whenever you are concerned, including when you hear rumors. Make sure they understand the consequences for the violations being discussed.

- Follow school policies and procedures, including any athletic codes that apply. Notify administrators designated by the policy of the results of your investigation and the actions you plan to take. Complete any documentation that is required.

- If appropriate, talk to the athlete's parents. Follow school policies and athletic codes concerning notification of parents. You

"Create rules with your super-intendent's daughter in mind, the starting center on your basketball team who has her first—and only—beer at the beginning of her senior year. If you can enforce the rule with her, it's probably fair for everyone."

Roger Svendsen, Minnesota Institute of Public Health

may be the right person to talk to the parents, or someone else in the school might be more suitable. In some cases, notification of the parents may not be necessary or appropriate.

- Apply consequences if there is sufficient evidence to show that a violation of the tobacco, alcohol, or other drug policy has oc-curred. A clearly written policy with reasonable consequences that have been previously communicated to athletes and their parents will make this process easier for everyone involved.

- Use this as a teachable moment for the individual athlete, the parents, and, when appropriate, for the entire team. Think ahead to the messages you want to convey. See chapter 5 for more in-formation on using teachable moments.

- Consider giving the athlete who has violated the policy the op-portunity to talk to the team. Balance the team's need for infor-mation with the need for privacy for the individual athlete.

- Reinforce positive behavior. In many situations there will be ath-letes who chose not to engage in inappropriate behavior or ath-letes who were honest with you while their teammates were dis-honest.

- If a violation has occurred, make a referral to the student assis-tance team or your key contact. See chapter 7 and Part III for information on using resources to back you up. Also, find ways to support the athlete who has violated the policy. This is also discussed in more detail in chapter 7.

- Be willing to take some risks. You may make errors in investigat-ing and in applying consequences, and athletes may choose to be dishonest with you. Few people bat 1.000. When a player lies to you and continues to play while teammates are honest and benched, the peer consequences may be worse than any suspen-sion you might give. You may not be perfect in enforcing policies, but these guidelines can help you be more consistent.

Rules Are Only a Small Part of Prevention

In spite of the fact that this chapter has been devoted entirely to this subject, codes of conduct and rules are a minor part of any preven-tion program. There is no perfect rule that will convince young people not to use. No rule or code fits every situation for all time. Any rule or code should be reviewed periodically, and groups affected by a given policy should have a voice in its creation. Athletic rules and codes need to be integrated with other organizational policies and programs. In any case, rules and codes are only one strategy for sending clear and consistent messages. As we discussed in chapter 2, athletes rarely say that a rule is the primary reason for their choice not to use to-bacco, alcohol, and other drugs.

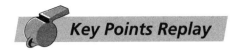

Key Points Replay

■ Remember, the purpose of rules is to help everyone—coaches, athletes, and parents—make good decisions.

■ Design your rules by keeping in mind the "good kid" who makes a mistake. Make sure consequences are fair and reasonable, and allow an athlete to recover from a mistake.

■ Enforce rules fairly and consistently. Apply the same consequences to all players for similar behaviors.

■ Do not ignore possible rule violations, even if the information comes to you as a rumor.

■ Work with your colleagues to enforce rules consistently among teams.

■ Use multiple opportunities to communicate rules to athletes and their parents throughout the season.

■ There is no perfect rule. Rules are only one part of prevention. Other prevention strategies are probably more effective than rules or laws.

Chapter

5

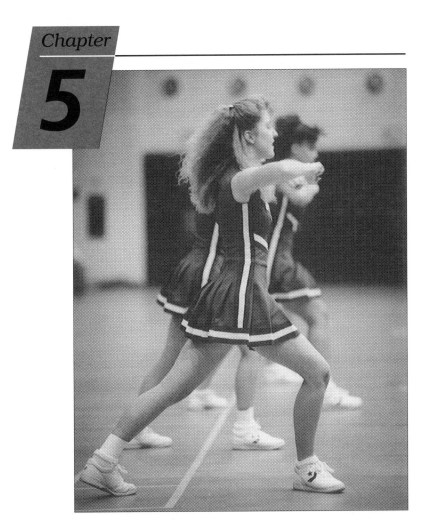

Using Opportunities to Teach

Chapter Warm-Up

Chapter 5 will help you use informal and formal opportunities to give information about tobacco, alcohol, and other drugs. You will be able to use multiple opportunities to counteract messages that promote the use of tobacco, alcohol, and other drugs. You will be able to conduct preseason meetings as one method of formally reaching parents and young people, and you will be able to recognize and use informal teachable moments throughout the year.

Research About Drug Education

Schools have been in the business of drug education for over 100 years. But it was not until the mid-1970s that research began to show which approaches worked—and which did not—to prevent problems with tobacco, alcohol, and other drugs. One of the strategies that has been closely evaluated is providing information about tobacco, alcohol, and other drugs.

Prevention research has not shown that programs that depend solely on providing information about health, social, and legal risks of tobacco, alcohol, and other drug use are effective. Information about drugs does not appear to be sufficient, but it is probably still necessary. Providing accurate information in combination with other strategies can result in measurable changes in attitudes and behavior.

As a coach, you will have numerous opportunities to provide information to athletes about tobacco, alcohol, or other drugs. As shown in Figure 5.1, there are nine factors you should keep in mind (adapted from Harding, Ringhofer & Associates, Inc., 1994).

- Be confident of your expertise.

- Be willing to talk about both sides of the issue.

- Create active learners.

- Be one of many messengers.

- Avoid mixed messages.

- Concentrate on short-term consequences.

- Avoid scare tactics.

- Use data cautiously.

- Use repetition.

Figure 5.1   Nine ways to get your message across.

Be Confident of Your Expertise

Research has shown that the credibility of the person giving information is significantly related to a young person's willingness to accept the messages given. Simply put, if young people believe the presenter is credible, they are more likely to believe what the presenter says. Research seems to indicate that an outside expert is not necessary in communicating about sensitive issues such as tobacco, alcohol, or other drug use. Other factors—such as familiarity to students, trustworthiness, or attractiveness—may be more significant. Coaches often have these characteristics in their relationships with young people; thus coaches can be powerful messengers. Because of the relationship you have with your athletes, your opinion may be more important to them than extensive factual information. You may not have the latest information on the newest drug, but when young people know that you think drugs are risky and dangerous to them and that you care about them, they may not need more information.

"The Reference Guide to Common Drugs" found in Appendix B gives information on the drugs young athletes most commonly use. In general, these drugs produce the following effects:

- They affect the central nervous system and other body systems.

- They affect the user's feelings, perceptions, mood, and judgment.

- They affect the user's behavior and motor coordination.

- They can interfere with normal growth and development.

- They can produce a psychological and physical dependence in which users may become dependent upon the effects of the drug and experience loss of control over their use. The cause of this dependency is not yet clearly known, and it is probably a combination of hereditary, physical, emotional, psychological, social, and environmental factors. Dependency can foster loss of motivation and the inability to handle responsibilities at school, on the job, or in personal relationships.

- They are implicated in many other serious problems affecting young people, including violence; teen pregnancy; HIV/AIDS and other sexually transmitted diseases; highway deaths, drownings, and other accidents; depression and suicide; child abuse; rape, including date rape; poor academic performance; and theft, vandalism, and other crimes against property.

- Illicit drugs carry special risks because their purity and dosage are usually unknown. Similar drugs may be sold in place of the real drug, or a drug may be cut with other substances. Effects can vary greatly. The manner in which illicit drugs are sold, bought, and used adds numerous other risks.

Be Willing to Talk About Both Sides of the Issue

Research has shown that two-sided messages are more effective than one-sided messages. A one-sided message concentrates on only the negative effects of tobacco, alcohol, and other drugs and ignores any potential benefits of their use. For example, athletes who are only exposed to information about the negative side effects of steroid use may be unprepared to counteract the information they get from their friends or other sources about the possible benefits. In fact, young people and their friends may experience positive benefits from drug use—at least initially. If the information about the benefits seems to be true, the provider of the one-sided message about the negative effects may lose credibility with the athlete.

Create Active Learners

The athlete's role in learning the information is also important. As with any other subject, active learning about tobacco, alcohol, and other drugs is far superior to passive learning. Young people need and want opportunities to talk about tobacco, alcohol, and other drugs with adults they trust. They do not generally want more factual information or another lecture about tobacco, alcohol, and other drugs. Rather, they want to talk and discuss situations they or their friends may be facing. As a coach, you can provide those opportunities.

Be One of Many Messengers

As we have said previously, multiple sources are superior to a single source. When young people hear the same positive messages from several sources—their friends, their parents, classroom teachers, coaches, other school activity staff, clergy, law enforcement personnel, and other significant adults—they are more likely to accept the message.

Avoid Mixed Messages

In chapter 3 we discussed how easy it is to give mixed messages about tobacco, alcohol, and other drugs. Young people get different messages about tobacco, alcohol, and other drugs from various sources, and sometimes they get different messages from the same source. For example, some schools have invited sports heroes who are ex-users to speak to young people. The message is often mixed. The speaker verbally encourages young people to not use tobacco, alcohol, and other drugs. Yet the athlete achieved success while using drugs and, even now, gains attention by telling stories of drug use. If we use such heroes in our prevention efforts, we should be aware of this message and balance it with equally attractive sports heroes who have chosen not to use.

Concentrate on Short-Term Consequences

Young people respond better to information about short-term consequences than long-term ones. For instance, young people are more likely to avoid smoking because of bad breath than because of the potential for lung cancer. They may also be more likely to avoid steroid use because of acne than potential heart disease. The long-term consequences of tobacco, alcohol, and other drug use usually happen when people are older, and most young people do not think that far into the future.

Avoid Scare Tactics

Approaches that attempt to scare young people away from a particular behavior do not seem to have any long-term impact. The aura of infallibility that surrounds most adolescents, particularly athletes, protects them from believing that anything bad could ever happen to them. Athletes generally have strong, healthy bodies and do not imagine themselves ever being sick or injured. Many adolescents watch their peers use—or use themselves—without apparent consequences. In this case, scare tactics only serve to discredit the presenter of the information.

Use Data Cautiously

Young people tend to believe and act on the misperception that "everybody is doing it." Promote, instead, the fact that most young people choose not to use tobacco, alcohol, and other drugs. Use trend data that clearly show how tobacco, alcohol, and other drug use has declined. (See Figure 1.1, p. 11. Trend data may also be available from your state department of education or from your local school district.)

Use Repetition

Sixty one-minute messages are better than an hour-long lecture.

Advertisers have long known that our behavior as consumers is strongly influenced by hearing and seeing brief, captivating commercials that are repeated many times. You can emulate this strategy by taking advantage of teachable moments to send brief, positive messages about not using tobacco, alcohol, and other drugs. (See "A Case for Repetition" in chapter 11.)

Informal Opportunities: Teachable Moments

Messages promoting the use of tobacco, alcohol, and other drugs are pervasive in our society. Although some messages are direct, most are subtle. These subtle messages suggest that drug use is associated with fame, fortune, or success in athletics or other pursuits. Often these messages promote both use and misuse of drugs, including underage consumption of tobacco and alcohol.

Often alcohol use is linked with athletic participation. According to a report of a study sponsored by the American Automobile Association Foundation for Traffic Safety, $1.7 billion was spent in 1990 on sports marketing (Wallack, Cassady, & Grube, 1990). The top two sponsors are two giants in the alcohol beverage industry, which each spent more than $60 million on special events in 1989, most of it on sporting events. In 1995, advertisers spent about $1 million for 30 seconds of advertising during the Super Bowl. These messages reach a large number of young viewers. The average American youth will see literally thousands of beer commercials before reaching the legal minimum drinking age. Sports programs contain approximately eight beer commercials per event. In addition, sports programming uses prime locations for banners, billboards, and other forms of promotion.

You cannot shelter young people from all messages that promote the use of tobacco, alcohol, and other drugs, nor can you necessarily sever the connections made between drug use and athletics.

We need many messengers to carry the same message.

However, you can challenge these messages by capturing the informal opportunities you have in your normal, day-to-day interaction with your players. As a coach, you are frequently confronted with situations that involve tobacco, alcohol, and other drugs. These situations range from close, personal times when young people confide in you, to situations involving groups of young people, to opportunities for counteracting larger societal messages. All are teachable moments. By thinking ahead, you can formulate the messages you want to send when these opportunities occur. Remember, the messages you send can be brief.

Here are a few examples of teachable moments and messages that can be sent to counteract pervasive pressures to use tobacco, alcohol, and other drugs.

Teachable Moments

- Team members violate rules about tobacco, alcohol, and other drugs. You talk to your team about the team rule, why you have a rule that prohibits the use of drugs, and how you feel about the rule and its violation.
- You hear rumors of an upcoming party. You talk about team commitment and discuss ways to have fun without alcohol or other drugs.
- A newspaper article features an athlete who was arrested for drug use. You discuss some of the consequences of drug use and concepts of role modeling.
- A television broadcast shows athletes celebrating victory with champagne. You talk to team members about celebrations and send the message that alcohol is not essential to celebrate.
- An athlete makes an unpopular choice not to go to a drinking party. You reinforce the choice and talk about pressure to use tobacco, alcohol, and other drugs.
- An athlete brings you an advertisement for a performance-altering drug or a nutritional supplement. You talk about the reliability of advertising and the importance of a good diet and a well-designed exercise and weight-training program.

Preseason Meetings: Building a Prevention Team

Many coaches throughout the country have found that preseason meetings are a great way to involve parents in their programs. Because athletics generally draw more parents than most other school-related events, preseason meetings provide one of the most effective means to reach and involve parents in athletics and prevention.

One of the strongest correlates of low use or nonuse of tobacco, alcohol, and other drugs is perception of parental concern: Those young people who believe that their parents would be upset if they

In Manhattan Middle School, Kansas, parent meetings are held before the beginning of each sport season. Discussions are held regarding the expectations coaches have of athletes and vice versa. Parent meetings offer parents information about prevention skills and activities, creating a parent network that can continue throughout high school.

On TARGET, February 1992

used are less likely to use than young people who think their parents wouldn't be concerned. This correlation holds as they get older. Both 8th graders and high school seniors who believe that their parents would be concerned are less likely to use than their peers. However, the numbers of young people who believe their parents would be upset decline dramatically from 8th to 12th grade. As young people move away from home, the perception of parental concern probably drops even further.

You can increase the chance that your athletes are getting clear nonuse messages from their parents by giving parents information about their important role in prevention, by presenting them with ideas for taking preventive action, and by encouraging and supporting their involvement in prevention.

However, involving parents may not be a selling point. Your experience with parents may have been unpleasant because of armchair quarterbacking or constant complaints. Yet this may be the very reason that parents should be involved. Many parents are probably supportive of your efforts but are in the silent majority. Their presence in a preseason meeting provides them with an opportunity to show their support and may silence some of the more negative parents. Preseason meetings offer an excellent opportunity to clear the air and resolve some of the concerns that may trouble parents.

General Topics

Preseason meetings provide everyone involved in athletics, including coaches, athletes, and their parents, an opportunity to openly discuss a variety of issues. Through preseason meetings, parents and activity participants get the information they need about activities, and they talk about rules and expectations. These are the topics most often included in a preseason meeting:

- Program philosophy
- Schedules
- Participation requirements
- Codes of conduct
- Participation fees
- Insurance
- Injury notification
- Team selection criteria

Athletic Training and Healthy Lifestyle Topics

Preseason meetings can also disseminate information about achieving optimal performance and health through

- proper nutrition,
- exercise,
- strength training,
- practice,

- stress management, and
- not using tobacco, alcohol, or other drugs.

Formats and Methods

Preseason meetings are conducted in a variety of ways. There are three major formats:

- Multiple teams meeting together in a large group
- Individual team meetings
- A combination of multiple teams in a large group meeting and individual team sessions

Within these three formats, a variety of methods—including speakers, videos, panel discussions, or group discussions—may be used to cover the topics.

Planning Considerations

The following are some questions to consider as you plan a preseason meeting (adapted from Harding, Ringhofer & Associates, Inc., 1994).

Identify Your Audience

Who do you want to have involved? Coaches? Other school activity staff members? Other school faculty? Team members? Parents? Other community members? The press? Is the meeting going to be for multiple teams? For single teams?

Clarify Your Purpose and the Benefits of This Meeting

Why do you want to work with this group? Why should they take the time to attend this meeting? What benefits will they receive?

Write Your Objectives

What do you want your audience to know as a result of attending? How do you want them to feel? What do you want them to do after they leave?

Create Your Agenda

How are you going to accomplish these objectives? Have a speaker? Show a film? Have a discussion? Who will lead each part of the meeting? How much time does each person have? Will there be an opportunity for parents and players to meet the coach? (Figure 5.2 gives a sample agenda for a preseason meeting.)

Select Your Time and Place

When and where are you going to hold this meeting?

Memorandum

August 30, 1993	The eligibility policy states that to be eligible to participate in any student activity attendance at some meetings is necessary. August 30 is a required meeting for any student who plans to participate in any student activity during the 1993-94 school year (athletics, music, drama, speech, cheerleading, etc.) AND ONE PARENT. Roll will be taken.
Date/Time:	Monday, August 30, 1993 at 6:30 p.m. Please make no other commitments for this time and make work arrangements now. This date was also announced in our April 1993 newsletter.
Place:	Ogden Community High School Gym
Format: 6:30-7:15	Those planning to participate in any nonathletic activity (music, drama, speech) and a parent meet in the Auditorium.
7:30-8:30	All students planning to go out for an activity during the 1993-94 school year and one parent meet in the gym. Our guest speaker will be Mr. Rich Nielsen. Mr. Nielsen is not only a dynamic speaker, he is also a magician, a juggler, and a humorist. He combines these talents to provide a motivational, inspirational and entertaining program. Information on sportsmanship, the eligibility policy, and health and injury issues will also be presented.
8:30-9:15	Those planning to participate in football, volleyball, cross-country, cheerleading, winter/spring/summer sports AND ONE PARENT will meet in separate areas.

Fall athletic practices are set to begin August 19.

Figure 5.2   Sample preseason meeting agenda.

Reprinted with permission from materials used by Ogden Community High School, Ogden, IA.

Additional Hints

Here are some additional suggestions to help you hold a successful preseason meeting:

- We recommend that you make participation by parents mandatory: One parent or guardian must attend the preseason meeting for his or her child to participate in the sport. Although we would not necessarily eliminate an athlete from a squad if a parent did not attend (see below for options), mandatory meetings generally get the greatest attendance. People have to justify not coming rather than decide why they should come instead of doing other things. If you are uncomfortable with "mandatory," or it is not feasible, then use the word "expected," which will get the next best attendance result. Using soft words, such as "invited" or "welcomed," will dramatically decrease parental attendance. (Figure 5.3 is a sample letter written to parents.)

- Make provisions for parents who cannot attend to obtain information by another method. Some coaches videotape the

Everett Public Schools
Administration Building

September 27, 1995

Dear Parent/Guardian:

As part of our ongoing philosophy of bringing students, parents and the school system closer, the Everett High School Athletic Department will be conducting a mandatory "Meet the Coach" meeting for *all* athletes in all sports (Fall, Winter, Spring seasons) and parents/guardians (adult). The meeting will take place on Tuesday, October 5, 1995 in the Rockwood Auditorium at Everett High School. Registration will be at 6:45 p.m. and the meeting will last approximately two hours.

The purpose of this meeting is to clearly explain the rules, regulations, and policies that govern interscholastic athletics at Everett High School. It will give parents an opportunity to meet the coaches and become acquainted with their individual expectations and philosophies. It will also develop improved and open lines of communication from which the student athletes of Everett High School will benefit.

One of the topics to be discussed will be alcohol, tobacco, and other drugs as they relate to the student athlete. The school system has a major commitment to the development of substance abuse prevention programs. In order to do this, we need to have parent help and support. We look forward to your assistance and working more closely with you.

If you have a conflict, please contact the head coach of your student athlete's team.

Sincerely yours,

Superintendent of Schools

Principal

Director of Athletics

| Figure 5.3 | Sample program letter. |

Reprinted with permission of Everett Public Schools, Everett, MA; John J. DiBiaso, Jr., Head Football Coach.

Knights Against Drugs (Tyler Consolidated High School, Sistersville, West Virginia) presented a special segment at a preseason meeting as parents and student athletes learned the new athletic policies and procedures that govern athletic participation.

On TARGET, September, 1993

meeting, hold another meeting for those with schedule conflicts, or schedule individual sessions with parents.

• Provide options for athletes who do not live with their parents or whose parents simply will not attend under any circumstances. In addition to not wanting to eliminate these athletes from a team, we do not want them to stand out at the preseason meeting. Encourage these athletes to bring a trusted adult.

• Eliminate as many barriers as possible that could keep parents from attending. Consider offering a meal, providing babysitting services, or making transportation available if these are barriers in your community. Organized parent groups or high school student leaders can provide some of these services for you.

• Build in fun. Remember that one of the main reasons young people participate in athletics is to have fun. As you plan your agenda, think of creative ways you can make this meeting fun for parents as well as athletes.

• Check out your objectives, agenda, and activities with others whom you expect to attend—especially athletes, parents, and other coaches—before you notify everyone.
• Suggest ways parents can get involved and provide a sign-up sheet in their information packet.

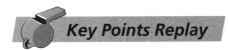

Key Points Replay

■ There are many situations concerning sports and drugs that arise naturally during the course of a season. Preparing for these situations allows us to use them as teachable moments.

■ Accurate information about tobacco, alcohol, and other drugs can be effective when combined with other prevention strategies. It is a necessary, but not sufficient, prevention strategy.

■ Using teachable moments may be the most effective method of providing information about tobacco, alcohol, and other drugs.

■ Because of your relationship with your athletes, your opinion is as important as factual information about tobacco, alcohol, and other drugs.

■ Preseason meetings are one of the best opportunities to reach parents with positive prevention messages. In addition, there are many other benefits of conducting preseason meetings.

■ Young people who perceive that their parents would be concerned about their use of tobacco, alcohol, and other drugs are less likely to use than their peers. As a coach, you can encourage your athletes' parents to share their concern.

6

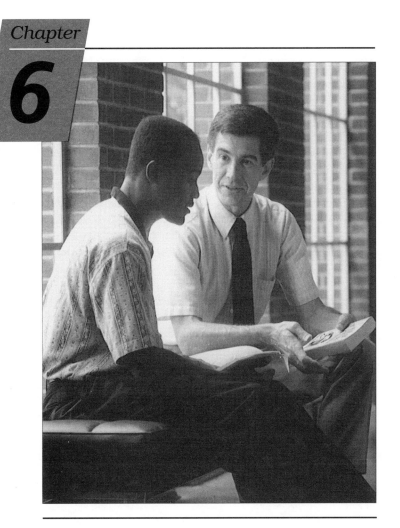

Involving Athletes and Parents in Prevention

Chapter Warm-Up

Chapter 6 will help you identify many additional strategies to prevent problems with tobacco, alcohol, and other drugs through athletics, such as student leadership training, parent networks, and parent-sponsored after-event parties. You will learn how you can be instrumental in getting parents and athletes involved because they are often the most appropriate people to carry out these strategies.

Why Involve Student Athletes in Prevention?

In Hutchinson, Kansas, 26 team members visit elementary and middle schools. They answer questions from the students about drugs and high school. "This is to let them know there are students who make a commitment not to use alcohol and drugs," said Randy Norwood, Hutchinson activities director.

On TARGET, January, 1991

Chapter 5 talked about the importance of parents in preventing tobacco, alcohol, and other drug use. Peers also play highly significant roles in the choices their friends and teammates make. Prevention research has shown that young people tend to use tobacco, alcohol, and other drugs in much the same way as their friends. Also, young people often turn to their friends for help and for information about tobacco, alcohol, and other drugs. By providing accurate information, setting appropriate standards, and presenting opportunities for young people to become involved in prevention, you can strengthen team members' commitment to nonuse and create more positive peer role models.

As previously discussed in chapter 1, team standards are often adopted by the team members. For instance, if sportsmanship is a standard that is valued by the leaders of the team, the members of the team will often adopt that standard or value. If sportsmanship is not valued by the team's leaders, the members are more likely to adopt unsportsmanlike behavior. If the captains of the soccer team have become known among student athletes for hosting drinking parties, it may be difficult for individual team members to choose not to drink. If the captains are drug free, others may follow their lead.

Leadership Training

One successful prevention strategy is to provide leadership training and ongoing support in order to help captains (and other leaders of athletic teams) be a positive influence for others on their team. Athletes often find themselves in leadership positions because of how other people view them. Captains of teams are often selected because of their seniority, physical skill, or popularity among their teammates. Those who select a captain often have high expectations. Yet in most situations, these expectations are not directly communicated.

Student leadership workshops can help captains and other team leaders explore and develop their leadership skills, including skills to handle situations involving tobacco, alcohol, and other drug use. Encouraging athletes to obtain specialized training is not a new strategy. Athletes are often encouraged to attend programs to develop their skills in a particular sport. Attending leadership training may be as beneficial to a captain as further developing athletic skills. The leadership skills they develop may be used in many ways, both in and outside of athletics.

You may not be directly involved in organizing, sponsoring, or even chaperoning such leadership training. As a coach, you can seek out these opportunities and attend workshops with your captains or other team leaders. You can also encourage your athletes to get involved in programs, activities, and leadership groups in the school and community.

Student Leader Efforts

Currently, there are four major approaches to involving student leaders in preventing problems with use of tobacco, alcohol, and other drugs. Each approach has a slightly different focus and group of students who are selected to participate. Athletes may be involved in any one of these four approaches. As we progress through this section, we will be primarily discussing the first option; the rest are given to distinguish these from leadership efforts that primarily involve the leaders of your teams or groups.

Team-Group Leadership

The focus of this approach is to ask student and adult leaders to work through their existing teams to prevent problems and promote healthy lifestyles. Students selected may be titled leaders, or they may be viewed as having high leadership potential within their sport. The training they receive helps them identify their leadership strengths, improve their leadership skills, and openly discuss issues, such as use of tobacco, alcohol, and other drugs, they may face as team leaders.

Peer Education/Peer Mentors

In this approach, student leaders (with adult support) work with same-age or younger students to provide structured educational programs to prevent problems and promote healthy lifestyles. Students selected are recognizable and visible leaders who make a strong commitment to the lifestyle behavior they are advocating. These peer educators or mentors become credible messengers about the standards and values we hope other young people will adopt. They also provide positive encouragement for younger children to become involved in athletics and other school activities. Training these student leaders provides a structure for their classroom sessions and encouragement for participating in this special effort. Athletes are an important element of any peer education program because of their visibility and popularity in schools. (See "Prevention Actions for Athletes and Their Parents: Cross-Age Education" on pp. 74-75 for more ideas.)

Peer Helping

In this approach, student leaders are a bridge between troubled students and helping services within the school and community. Students and adults who are selected are viewed as good listeners and viable sources of help to other students and adults within the school. A broad mix of students is chosen to represent different school factions. Athletes are an important part of any peer-helping program because they can reach the athletic segment of the school community. The training they receive helps them learn good communication and helping skills and become familiar with the helping resources within the school and community.

Special Action Groups

Many schools also have student-led groups whose sole focus is to solve a particular problem. Students Against Driving Drunk (SADD) may be the best known of these groups, but there are many other local, state, regional, and national groups that encourage students to be active in prevention. The membership of these groups is usually determined by the interest of the students themselves; there is usually no formal selection process. National organizations may offer training that teaches students organizational skills to accomplish their specific tasks.

Leadership Training Opportunities

There are many sources of leadership training opportunities for your athletes. The following are a few you should consider.

State or Regional Training

"At Pleasant Grove High [Utah] we have trading cards for the school's sports teams to promote being drug free. The players on the cards, of course, must be drug free. Kids at all schools really look up to the sports players. They want to be like them. If these players are drug free, then they set a good example."

Jenni Fisher
On TARGET,
December, 1992

State athletic or activity associations often sponsor training for student leaders, holding it at regional or central locations. Usually schools are allowed to send only a few students with their adult coaches or sponsors. This option gives young people and adults the opportunity to share ideas and strategies with each other. Seeing that others have experienced similar problems—and achieved success in resolving them—can motivate adults and young athletes to take action.

Conference or District Training

Sometimes athletic leagues or conferences (or districts, sections, or regions) will sponsor training for student and adult leaders in their member schools. Individual schools send a few students and adults who have the opportunity to interact with athletes with whom they compete. This has the additional potential of improving sportsmanship within the district or conference.

Sometimes, large school districts with multiple high schools will pool their resources and provide training for several schools' athletic programs within their city.

Local, One-School Training

This option can provide a school district with the opportunity to train the largest number of students and adults. Often this training will encompass the student leadership of a variety of teams and groups within the school and can help to foster cooperation and unity among these groups. This option may have a greater impact on shaping the values and attitudes of a larger number of students within a school.

School districts may focus on particular leaders, such as the designated captains of teams and groups, with the expectation that they choose not to use tobacco, alcohol, and other drugs. Captains are given the option to step down if they choose not to fulfill this part of their responsibility. These schools also provide ongoing support to help these leaders live up to the expectations placed on them.

Providing Ongoing Support

Regardless of the option chosen for training or the types of leadership groups in which students are involved, adults need to provide support and follow-up in the school environment. Leadership support groups can provide an ongoing forum for captains or other team leaders to refine their leadership skills, solve problems, and get support for issues and stresses that they have in common. Support groups can also help captains (and all athletes) maintain their commitment to being drug-free. Some of these groups may limit membership to athletes or other young people involved in school activities; some may be open to broader membership.

Prevention Actions for Athletes and Their Parents

The preceding information has proposed several important ways to involve student athletes and their parents in prevention. Chapter 5 discussed the importance of preseason meetings. This chapter has concentrated on leadership training and ongoing leadership support groups. The following are additional actions that many parents and athletes are taking throughout the country. You may choose to initiate some of these actions on behalf of your athletes and their parents. Many of these efforts can—and should—be sponsored and led by the parents and students themselves. Many reach beyond your athletic program and into the community. However, your encouragement can be pivotal.

Voluntary Pledges

In Fayette County Public Schools, Kentucky, the Athletes Taking Action program encourages athletes to take a stand against tobacco, alcohol, and other drug abuse by accepting and wearing a patch.

On TARGET, May, 1990

Signing a pledge not to use tobacco, alcohol, and other drugs during the season is one strategy used to encourage athletes to make a commitment to nonuse. These pledges are often printed statements which describe why it is important for athletes to not use tobacco, alcohol, and other drugs, and the pledges stipulate that the athlete's signature is an agreement not to use. Figure 6.1 shows the Iowa State High School Athletic Association's voluntary pledge.

Signing voluntary pledges not to use tobacco, alcohol, or other drugs can reinforce the commitment of those athletes who are already committed to nonuse. Voluntary pledges may also encourage some athletes who occasionally use to stop using during the season. However, even if signing pledges is voluntary, some athletes will sign because they believe they have no choice if they want to play or be a part of the team. Others may sign because they believe it will be tantamount to admitting that they use tobacco, alcohol, or other drugs if they do not sign. Usually these athletes are in the minority. The entire effort

PLEDGE TO BE ALCOHOL AND DRUG FREE

I, —————————————————,
do hereby pledge to myself, my teammates, my
school, and to the Iowa High School Athletic
Association, that I will not use alcohol or drugs
during the ————————————— Season.

Signed this ——————— *day of*
————————————, 19———

——————————————————————
Student Signature

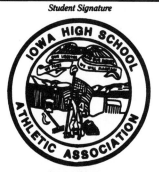

IOWA HIGH SCHOOL ATHLETIC ASSOCIATION
Boone, Iowa 50036   0991

Figure 6.1   Pledge to be alcohol and drug free.

Reprinted with permission of Iowa High School Athletic Association, Boone, IA.

"We know our youth are a tremendous resource. We hope to enlist and empower one segment of the school, those participating in athletics and activities. We hope they will become ambassadors for a drug-free lifestyle in their schools and show the leadership required to achieve this."

Des Jones, prevention specialist, Lake County, Grayslake Illinois. On TARGET, November, 1990

should not be scrapped just because a few athletes may choose to be dishonest.

Just like any of the suggestions that we have described, this strategy is not foolproof. It does, however, help to set a standard, and it may encourage many athletes to choose not to use. If you decide to use voluntary pledges, here are some suggestions:

- Use the opportunity to present the pledge as a time to talk to the team about tobacco, alcohol, and other drug use.
- Do not require athletes to sign the cards in the presence of other team members. This type of pressure may cause athletes to make a commitment that they have no intention of keeping.
- Explain the pledge to the athletes. Ask them to take their pledge, sign it, and return it to you at a designated time. Or ask them to return the card to the athletic director or another school staff member in order to eliminate any beliefs a player may have about your attitude toward those who choose or do not choose to sign the pledge.
- Use every opportunity to recognize those who choose to sign the pledge. Some schools publicly display the pledges or a list of those who have signed. Consider offering T-shirts, emblems, or other tangible incentives for signing.
- Understand that there are athletes who will not live up to their commitment. Use those tough times as teachable moments with the athlete. After all, many adults do not live up to the commitments they make. (Iowa High School Athletic Association, 1993)

Team Meetings

Team meetings are held by athletes to discuss a variety of issues, including tobacco, alcohol, and other drugs. These meetings are often led by the team captains, without coaches present. Standards of behavior are established by team members, and actions taken for violations of these standards are discussed. The purpose of these meetings is to develop a consensus or a solid base of support about appropriate and inappropriate behavior concerning tobacco, alcohol, and other drugs.

These standards and actions may not be identical to the rules and consequences for rule violations. For instance, team members may agree not to use tobacco, alcohol, and other drugs during the season but not agree about the rest of the year. They may not agree that "guilt by association" is appropriate. However, the team is more likely to have ownership of standards they develop than rules that they had no part in creating. The standards developed in this manner will probably be in closer agreement with the school's athletic policies than if no standards are discussed and individual team members are left to make their own decisions about whether or not to follow these policies.

The actions taken by team members to address those who violate team standards are understandably limited. Athletes, including captains, generally do not want to become rule enforcers. Captains may talk to a team member the first time a teammate violates the standard, thus giving the violator a "second chance." After such a warning, the captains may decide to go to the coach with additional violations by the team member. The team also may not agree on any action to take if a team member violates the team's agreements. Yet having some established standards (and a discussion on those standards) at least gives athletes more of an opportunity to talk to team members about behavior that the athletes believe is inappropriate. Regardless of the actions that your team leaders take, you may still need to enforce aspects of the athletic code or school policy that the team has not accepted, discussed, or agreed upon.

For this strategy to be successful, team captains must be thoroughly trained, have a strong, personal commitment to nonuse, and be given ongoing support. You must be confident in their leadership abilities—their willingness to stand up for their beliefs, their ability to communicate clearly with teammates, their level of respect for their teammates, and the level of respect their teammates have for them. You must be confident in their willingness to communicate with you about their leadership concerns, including those about tobacco, alcohol, and other drug use. You also need a certain amount of faith in the approach of building compliance through consensus.

Cross-Age Education

In Athletes Against Drugs, a Kingston School, New York, program, high school athletes speak to elementary classrooms in order to spread the message that drugs and sports do not mix. Older students set the example of how to say "no" for younger students.

On TARGET, May, 1991

Speaking to younger students about sports and the importance of choosing not to use tobacco, alcohol, and other drugs can be another way to involve athletes in prevention. Cross-age education is effective not only in helping the younger student not to use tobacco, alcohol, or other drugs but also in reinforcing this commitment in older athletes. When athletes speak to younger students about not using tobacco, alcohol, and other drugs, it is important for the athlete to make a firm commitment to being drug-free. The credibility of the whole effort can be jeopardized if the athlete is using and the younger students find out. Athletes who have used in the past, but have since stopped, can be included in these efforts because they can have an important message to send to the younger students. As we discussed in chapter 5, inviting recovering, chemically dependent students to speak to younger students may send a mixed message. Athletes with a brief history of nonuse (sobriety) are also at risk of relapse. Typically, a period of sobriety of at least six months to one year should occur before using athletes in this manner. If recovering athletes are used in this way, it is vitally important to balance their presentations with students who have chosen to not use tobacco, alcohol, and other drugs.

Training, resources and materials, and adult support are vital to adequately prepare athletes and other young people who are involved in these programs. Some athletes may have an easy time talking about nonuse of tobacco, alcohol, and other drugs, but it may be difficult for others. All athletes benefit from a structure that will allow them to more fully participate in cross-age education. In addition, the efforts are likely to fit better with other prevention strategies and be more beneficial to the younger students. *Everyone a Hero*, developed by the Colorado High School Activities Association, is one example of a structured program that provides a consistent format for athlete cross-age education (Harding, Ringhofer & Associates, Inc., 1992).

Preseason Meetings

Parents and athletes can help sponsor or conduct preseason meetings to make sure they are fun, informative, and organized to meet the needs of those who attend. If a key element in prevention through athletics is to have athletic directors, coaches, parents, and athletes working together, why not have all these groups involved in leading preseason meetings? Parents can help with letters and announcements to recruit other parents, food, transportation, or childcare services. Parents can also talk about their involvement in aftergame or event activities, parent networks, and other ways parents can be involved in prevention. Athletes can help in recruiting parents to the preseason meeting and assist parents with some of the arrangements mentioned above. Athletes can talk about how tobacco, alcohol, and other drug use affects the team and why it is important not to use. Some schools have team captains publicly state that they do not use tobacco, alcohol, and other drugs and why they think it is important not to use.

Aftergame Parties

Parents or athletes can host aftergame parties to provide a fun event where tobacco, alcohol, and other drugs are not used. Aftergame events and contests are often high-risk times for athletes. Athletes are usually still feeling the effects of their earlier competition. Adrenaline levels may still be high. They may be excited about doing well or depressed about doing poorly. Many athletes look forward to the time after games to spend time with their teammates and relax after the event. Aftergame parties give athletes, coaches, and parents an opportunity to get together in an environment that does not encourage the use of tobacco, alcohol, or other drugs.

Encourage team members' parents to organize food and activities for these events. In most schools, parties are not scheduled on nights when students have school the next day or if a party would conflict with other school events, such as dances, concerts, or fundraising events. Parents and athletes conduct a variety of activities at these parties, making sure that they offer low-stress activities. Athletes enjoy watching videos of earlier games or contests. Parties are more successful when athletes have input about what type of activities they would like to include. In some communities, parents and athletes may host these events at their homes; in others, they may work together to sponsor these events at the school or in other community buildings.

Activities With Competing Schools

Encourage parents and athletes to sponsor dances and other activities with competing schools. These mixers can provide fun, drug-free events and promote sportsmanship. Similar to aftergame or event parties, these activities add a twist by including the other team. They generally follow games or contests at the same site. However, other times and locations may be preferable.

Positive Promotional Materials

Athletes can help create T-shirts, buttons, flyers, or other materials that promote athletics and discourage the use of tobacco, alcohol, and other drugs. This can be a means of spreading the message of nonuse to other young people. Because many athletes are often watched by others and may be role models, wearing a T-shirt or button promoting nonuse may be seen by many other young people. The items selected for the promotion should be something the athlete likes to wear or have. The message should also be one the athletes like, accept, and are willing to honor (and, of course, a message that you and your administration are willing to endorse). Get the athletes' involvement in helping to select the items and the message.

Public Service Announcements

Another way for athletes to use their influence in reaching others is by broadcasting public service announcements. These announcements promote involvement in athletics and other positive activities and discourage the underage use of tobacco, alcohol, and other drugs. Athletes may create the announcements themselves or use ideas from national or state prevention organizations. Often, community radio or TV stations will give free air time for such announcements. The announcements can also be aired at games or contests and over the high school public address system.

Rules and Codes Revision

When creating, reviewing, or communicating information about rules or codes concerning the use of tobacco, alcohol, and other drugs, involve athletes and parents in the process. This can help reduce barriers to the acceptance of the rules. This group can play a vital role in representing various points of view and in communicating the rule and the process to other athletes and parents. This can increase the perception that there is general consensus about the rule and its consequences. (Chapter 4 further describes the process of developing and implementing rules and codes.)

Prevention Workshops

Just as athletes and parents can be involved in planning and conducting preseason meetings, they can also design, organize, and sponsor prevention workshops. Both parents and athletes can take part in these or other prevention workshops. We particularly recommend that any athletes or parents who are involved in rule-revision committees take part in a workshop with other committee members.

Parent Networks

"Parents, acting together, are changing community attitudes and are reducing teen drinking and other drug use and preventing sometimes tragic outcomes. It is not easy. It takes work. Parents are giving up a great deal of their leisure time to organize and promote community-wide networks. Other parents are agreeing to follow the same guidelines. That's what it takes."

Tom Walsh, Parents Communication Network, St. Paul, MN. On TARGET, November, 1990

Parent networks give parents a means to send a nonuse message about tobacco, alcohol, and other drugs to young people in the community. The primary focus of these networks is prevention. These networks are organized and run by a small number of parents, but they involve a large number of parents of athletes and nonathletes in the community. The only requirement for full membership in a parent network is to follow a set of simple guidelines that set a standard for parents. As members, parents may agree to (adapted from Blaszczak, 1992)

- sponsor only tobacco-, alcohol-, and other drug-free chaperoned events for their children at home or in the community;
- learn about parenting skills and other information related to tobacco, alcohol, and drug prevention and intervention;
- communicate a nonuse message and prevention information about tobacco, alcohol, and other drugs to their children;
- talk with other parents about where their children are going, with whom, whether or not an event is free of tobacco, alcohol, and other drugs, chaperoned, and if there is an appropriate curfew; and
- work with the network and within the school and community, whenever possible, to promote a unified approach to reducing tobacco, alcohol, and other drug use within the community.

In addition to communicating a nonuse message to young people, a parent network can organize drug-free events, such as aftergame and event parties and afterprom or graduation parties. Parents cut across all segments of the community. Having an organized parents group can aid in getting more segments of the community to send the same nonuse message to young people, including young athletes.

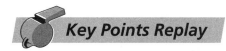

Key Points Replay

- Peers, as well as parents, play an important role in the choices that young people make about tobacco, alcohol, and other drugs.

- There are many strategies that parents and athletes can use to prevent tobacco, alcohol, and other drug use. These strategies help set a nonuse standard for adolescents, provide drug-free places for athletes to gather during high-risk times, and heighten the visibility of athletes and parents who are committed to prevention.

- Whatever strategies are chosen, young people should be involved in designing and implementing them.

■ The designated leaders of your teams do not always have the skills or knowledge to take a stand that promotes nonuse. Leadership training can help them be more effective in whatever leadership roles they choose to take in your school.

■ You can play a critical role in seeing that athletes on your team and their parents are involved in implementing many of the strategies discussed in this chapter.

7

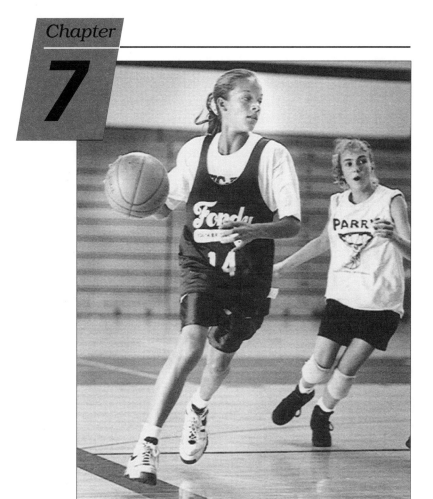

Responding Effectively

Chapter Warm-Up

Chapter 7 will help you respond more effectively when you become concerned about a student. You will define your legitimate role in responding to athletes and overcome many of the obstacles that may prevent you from responding. You will be better equipped to talk to athletes when you become concerned, and you will know the resources that are available to back you up. The following information will describe the role of the coach in responding to troubled athletes, and Part III will cover the function of a student assistance program in more depth.

Role of the Coach in Responding to Problems

As a coach, you are often in a good position to notice young people who are experiencing problems. Your professional training, work experience, and relationships with young people give you an edge in identifying these young people and creating an opportunity for them to receive the help they need.

The process described in this section can be used any time you are concerned about a young person. It is not problem specific. While it is helpful for identifying and responding to young people who are experiencing problems with tobacco, alcohol, and other drugs, it can be equally useful in helping young people who are in other kinds of trouble. This process does not require you to diagnose or label young people before you intervene. It simply counts on your ability to observe and identify behavior and then to directly and honestly share your concern. You can also use this process to give a young person positive feedback about performance or behavior.

Why Coaches Do Not Respond

As we have talked with coaches throughout the country, a clear picture has emerged about why coaches do not respond—even when they are aware that something is troubling an athlete.

Inadequate Training

Most colleges and universities do not provide training for teachers and coaches in responding to students who are experiencing problems. Teachers are usually prepared to handle classes of students, not to discuss personal problems with students. Consequently, coaches may feel unprepared to talk to an athlete about problems that are outside the realm of the sport. Many coaches now come to coaching from outside the school system and may feel even more unprepared to respond to troubled students. In addition to these factors, the role of the coach may not have been clearly defined. If coaches believe they are being asked to spot athletes who are having tobacco, alcohol, or other drug-use problems or to be adolescent counselors, they may rightfully feel they do not have the expertise to respond.

No Support

Some coaches simply are afraid to go out on a limb for fear they will not be supported by the school and community in getting help for an athlete. They may have had actual experience in referring an athlete for help, only to have nothing happen. They may be afraid that the community will not have the necessary resources to help the athlete. If coaches do not teach in the school building, they may be unfamiliar with the procedures and programs that are available to back them up.

Fear of Reaction

Talking to someone about personal concerns is always a risky business. Some coaches are afraid that students or parents will react in anger or expect them to solve the problems. Sometimes it is easier to just avoid the whole subject than to bring it up and risk a negative reaction. Some coaches may fear lawsuits, feeling that, if they overstep their bounds, the parents will sue them or the school.

Lack of Time

For some coaches, not responding to student problems is a matter of not having enough time. Caught among work, family, and social obligations, these coaches just do not feel they can take the time to adequately address a student's problems.

Because of the close relationship of coaches to young athletes, not responding can give the wrong impression. When we fail to respond, young people often interpret our lack of response incorrectly. One interpretation says we do not care about them: "The coach just doesn't care about anything except how well I can play." Another interpretation says their behavior is appropriate: "The coach didn't say anything about it, so we thought it was all right."

The approach that will be described in the following pages allows coaches to respond to athletes in a way that does not require extensive training or take tremendous time. It is an approach that is legally defensible, in that it fits cleanly into a coach's job. And it reduces the chance that parents or students will react negatively.

Five Aspects of Your Role

This section will examine five aspects of responding to troubled students that are well within your legitimate role as a coach (Figure 7.1). The materials in this section are adapted from the TARGET Leadership Training Manual (Harding, Ringhofer & Associates, Inc., 1994).

> - Observing and identifying behavior
> - Sharing concern
> - Upholding expectations
> - Providing support
> - Referring

Figure 7.1   Five guidelines for responding to troubled students.

Observing and Identifying Behaviors

The first step is to observe and identify behavior that causes you to be concerned about a young person. In your job as a coach, you spend countless hours with young people, watching them participate in cocurricular activities, attend classes, or take part in other organized activities. In addition to these structured hours, you probably also see them during times they think they are not being observed: in the hallways, in your community, or talking with their friends. The sheer amount of time you spend with young people gives you a unique vantage point to observe their behavior. You also have a perspective on adolescence that allows you to notice when something is out of the ordinary. Plus, your coaching skills can help you out. You are used to watching an athlete's performance and giving specific feedback on how to maintain and improve that performance; young athletes are used to getting feedback from you.

You are responsible for the process, not the outcome.

The behaviors that are out of the ordinary could be caused by a variety of problems: tobacco, alcohol, and other drug use; family conflict; divorce; exposure to violence; physical or sexual abuse; loss of a family member or close friend; the breakup of a personal relationship; physical problems; pregnancy; or any other of many problems that affect young people. However, the behaviors you observe may not always reflect an underlying problem. The young person may simply be trying out behaviors that are not appropriate.

In any case, it is not necessary to know what causes the behavior before you respond. In fact, attempting to diagnose the underlying cause can be counterproductive. It can delay your response time, it can lead to labeling a young person, and it is usually outside your legitimate role as a coach.

After noting the behaviors, it can be helpful to jot them down on a piece of paper before taking the next step: sharing your concern.

Sharing Concern

The process of sharing concern uses a series of "I" statements. This process attempts to avoid some of the major pitfalls in talking to students: blaming, judging, labeling, yelling, lecturing, accusing, preaching, assuming, embarrassing, demanding, and threatening. These "adultisms" frequently make it impossible for young people to hear what adults have to say. Young people may become so preoccupied with protecting themselves that they cannot listen and are unwilling to talk with adults. The process also allows you to slow down enough to think through the messages you want to send. It helps you be more positive in your approach to young people. Table 7.1 lists responses that young people have repeatedly given to us when we ask them how they would like their coaches to respond.

A Six-Step Process for Sharing Concern

The following section shows a structure for sharing our concern that will help us to take advantage of the athletes' suggestions on how coaches should respond to athletes.

Table 7.1 Student Preferences	
Do	**Do not**
Let me know you care	Lecture
Talk to me	Yell
Listen	Keep prying
Keep it confidential	Accuse
Give me choices	Blame
Pay attention	Judge
Follow through	Ignore
Be persistent	Threaten
Be respectful	Do it in front of other people
Find an appropriate time to talk	Label
Be sincere	Blab it all over
Get the whole story	Assume
Be encouraging and positive	Overreact
Ask for help from others	Give advice
Take me seriously	Tell me about when you were my age

Table 7.2 Alternatives for Communication	
Try saying	**Do not say**
You missed three practices.	You are not living up to your commitment.
You decreased your speed from . . . to	You are slacking off.
You do not look at me when I talk to you.	You are disrespectful.
You were late twice this week.	You are irresponsible.
You have different friends.	You are hanging out with the wrong kids.
You are doing the minimum number of	You are lazy; you are not giving 100%.
You yelled at the manager yesterday.	You are an angry person.
Your eyes are red.	What are you on, anyway? Drugs?

I Care . . . .   Let the athlete know that he is important to you and to the rest of the team or group. You may be comfortable telling him directly that you care about him, or you may let him know indirectly by a smile, a gesture, or by letting him know that he is important to the team.

I See . . . .   Focus on observable behavior. What tipped you off that something was wrong? What did you see or hear that caused you to be concerned in the first place? (See suggestions in Table 7.2.)

Focusing on observable behavior helps you avoid labeling, being judgmental, or accusing the athlete.

I Feel . . . .   Give the athlete the benefit of knowing how you feel about her behavior. Feelings are expressed in one word only: "I feel angry," or "I feel worried." This lets the athlete know that what she is doing is affecting someone else. It can also reduce the chance of raising defenses and getting into an argument.

Listen . . . .   Listen to what the athlete has to say. Ask questions. Pay attention to him by resisting other distractions. Use good non-verbal listening skills. Be prepared for silence. You have picked the time and place to talk about this issue. Recognize that he may not be prepared to talk at this time. Also be prepared for anger, a sad or tragic story, or an emotional outpouring. When confronted, most people do not just say "thank you" and immediately change their behavior.

I Want . . . .   Once you have heard her perspective, let her know what you would like to have happen. Do you want her to follow team expectations? Seek help? Talk to someone else? Stay on the team? This is an opportunity to reinforce your standards and to state how you want the behavior to change.

I Will . . . .   Then let the athlete know how you will provide support. What are you willing to do? Go with the athlete to seek help from someone else? Be available to talk at another time? This lets the athlete know that he is not alone. You have a stake and a role in helping him change. It can be very threatening to be asked to change behavior; your support can reinforce your bond with the athlete and make it possible for him to change.

> **EXAMPLE 1:**
>
> The following example shows how this process can be used when you are concerned about a particular behavior, have a good idea what the problem is, and want to avoid diagnosing or labeling.
>
> *Coach:* Hey, Scott!
>
> *Scott:* Coach?
>
> *Coach:* You're doing a great job this year. You're hitting the holes faster this year than last. I need to talk to you about something.
>
> I watched you in practice today and noticed you were spitting a lot. Your jeans have a ring worn on the back pocket. When I've been standing next to you, I thought I smelled tobacco. I'm worried about you, Scott.
>
> *Scott:* There's nothing to worry about, coach. You've gotta spit with those mouth guards in. I put an empty can in my pocket to get that ring. Everybody's got one. And tobacco? My parents smoke, and I just can't get it out of my clothes.
>
> *Coach:* But I'm talking about when you're in your practice uniform, on the field.

When confronted, most people do not just say 'thank you' and immediately change their behavior.

Scott: Must've been somebody else.

Coach: So you are telling me that you don't chew tobacco.

Scott: That's right, coach.

Coach: That's good. Because I'm sure you know how harmful chewing tobacco can be. We have a team rule about the use of chewing tobacco, because it isn't good for you. And we don't want our players giving that kind of an image of our school.

We have a two-game suspension for those who use, and I sure don't want to lose you. You're doing so good this year.

Scott: (Walks out the door without responding.)

Coach: Oh . . . by the way . . . I know how hard it is to quit chewing. I used to chew. But we have resources at this school to help kids quit. Let me know if you want to talk about this another time.

EXAMPLE 2:

The following example shows how the six-step process can be used when you are concerned about a student and do not know the underlying problem.

Coach: Jennifer, one of your teachers caught me in the hall this morning and asked me what I intended to do about your grades. She said you were going to be ineligible if you didn't pass her class this quarter.

Jennifer: I suppose that was Mrs. Erickson. She's just got it out for me. I can't do anything right in that class.

Coach: I believe it takes more than one bad grade to make you ineligible, Jen. You were late for practice twice last week, and I've noticed that you look tired.

Jennifer: So you've got it out for me, too, now?

Coach: No, I just want you to know that you're important to me, and to the team. We need you. Besides, I'm getting concerned about you. What's going on?

Jennifer: You just don't know what it's like. Nobody does. If you lived in my house, you'd miss practice and get lousy grades. I just can't do everything and please everybody.

Coach: Sounds like a lot of stress to me. What's up?

Jennifer: My mom lost her job, so now there's nobody working except me. I can't even make enough money to keep gas in my car much less pay the rent. So I'm working until closing now, trying to keep everything going.

Coach: You're right. A 17-year-old shouldn't be responsible for paying for the family's bills. And you've got your grades to think about. I think we should go talk to somebody else about this. Would you be willing to talk to Mr. Jackson?

Jennifer: I don't know. What can he do?

Coach: I'm not sure. But some kids have told me he's been able to help them. I'll go with you. How about fifth hour?

Jennifer: I suppose.

Coach: I'll get a pass for you and meet you in the hallway outside his office.

Hints for Sharing Concern

You do not have to follow the six-step process exactly; it simply helps you plan what you want to say ahead of time. And, as shown in these examples, it can help you keep on track. Use your own words and your own style when sharing your concern with an athlete. Here are a few additional hints:

1. Consider the time and place. Find a time you can speak in private.

2. Leave the door open. This may be your time to talk, but not the athlete's. Let the athlete know you would be willing to talk some other time.

3. You can share your concern positively and offer to help. However, the athlete is ultimately responsible for his behavior and for taking action to change it.

4. Know your limits. Find out who else in your organization can back you up. Make sure you get help if you think the person is being harmed or may be considering harming herself or someone else. Check out school policies and mandatory reporting requirements for staff members. Certain behaviors and information cannot be kept confidential between you and your athletes.

5. Avoid words and phrases that automatically blame, such as "should," "must," "have to," or "you've got to understand that." "I" statements lessen the feeling that you are blaming the athlete. Also avoid words that are general and global, such as "always," "never," "everyone," and "nobody."

Upholding Expectations

Part of your job as a coach is to help young people learn from their actions. You also have a responsibility to uphold the expectations you have for members of your teams. You can remind athletes of these expectations during the "I want" part of the sharing-concern process. Then you must follow through. You may be tempted not to pursue action if you find out that the athlete has a personal problem that is causing the behavior. In most cases, however, lowering expectations can be detrimental by teaching the athlete to avoid personal responsibility. When expectations like rules aren't upheld consistently, the impact on preventing future problems can be hampered (see chapter 4 for more information on enforcing rules fairly and consistently).

Providing Support

At the same time you uphold expectations, you can support young people in their struggles to make good choices. You can disapprove of the behavior without disapproving of the athlete. Keeping focused on the specific behaviors that caused you to be concerned can help you make this distinction. You provide support by letting them know you care about them, by listening to their concerns, by checking back with them at a later time, and by referring them to others who can be of further help. The "I will" part of the sharing-concern process allows you to verbally provide support. Your actions show how committed to providing support you actually are. Chapter 9 will give you more ideas about how you can show your support for athletes if it becomes necessary to refer them for ongoing help.

Referring

Although the young person has come to you for help, or you have chosen to share your concerns, you may not be the most appropriate person to help the young person resolve the problem. At times, the young person may be completely resistant to what you have to say and unwilling or unable to change behavior patterns. He may disclose a problem that is beyond your expertise or capability to help. You may be concerned about the immediate safety of the young person or her family and friends. At that time, it is important for you to use your influence to help the young person and the family to seek further help.

It is almost impossible for you, as a coach, to keep track of all of the resources available to help young people with the problems they may face. However, it is generally possible to find one person in a school or community who can function as a key contact. This key contact provides backup and support for you and finds appropriate help for the young athlete. In schools, this key contact may be an individual counselor, social worker, psychologist, nurse, or administrator. Many schools are fortunate to have an assistance program where all of these helping professionals work together in a systematic team approach. (Chapters 8, 9, and 10 will further describe this approach, let you know what you can expect from this process, and tell you how you can use it.)

For other coaches, this key contact can be a mental health professional, a member of the clergy, a health care professional, or an educator. As a coach, you can find one person who can function as a key contact for referral. Helpful characteristics in this key contact include the following:

The "I will" part of the sharing-concern process allows you to verbally provide support. Your actions show how committed to providing support you actually are.

- Knowledge about community resources for adolescents
- Able to provide broad-based assessment services (or have access to these services)
- Willing to support you in your efforts to help the young person
- Has good rapport with young people
- Can work with parents and other family members
- Is accessible
- Has no vested interest in the outcome of an assessment
- Has a good reputation in the community

Figure 7.2 shows a model of an assistance process from the time an athlete displays a behavior that causes you to be concerned.

Assistance Process

Staff member

Athletic director or
coach

**OBSERVES AND IDENTIFIES
BEHAVIOR
SHARES CONCERN
UPHOLDS EXPECTATIONS
PROVIDES SUPPORT
REFERS, IF APPROPRIATE**

Key contact

Student assistance team
or key contact

Accepts referrals
Communicates with young person,
  other staff, and parents
Gathers information
Makes a pre-assessment
Sets goals and develops a plan
Provides support
Refers to additional resources,
  if appropriate

**School or community
resource**

Continues assessment
Provides education,
  counseling, and treatment
Offers aftercare and other
  support

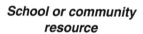 **Figure 7.2**   Assistance process emphasizing chapter 7 stages.
Adapted from Harding, Ringhofer & Associates, Inc., 1994.

Legal Issues in Responding

The courts have generally supported schools and individual staff members when they have acted in good faith on behalf of the student. They have been less supportive when schools or staff members failed to respond when it was apparent that a problem existed. In general, the courts examine the role of the school as an educational institution when making such determinations. If behaviors are interfering with the student's ability to participate fully in the educational process and, therefore, interfering in the school's ability to educate the child, then an intervention is legally appropriate. If the school is specific in identifying behavior that is interfering with the child's education and avoids diagnosing problems, then it is seen as staying within the boundaries of its educational mission.

Special Barriers for Athletes in Receiving Help

Chapter 1 described some of the special factors that may actually make some young athletes more susceptible to problems with tobacco, alcohol, and other drugs. Similar factors may also interfere with an athlete's ability to seek help or with others' ability to recognize problems when they occur.

Visibility

As we discussed in chapter 1, athletes are often visible in their communities and, therefore, are more vulnerable to criticism from many people. This visibility—and their fear of having personal problems discussed in the community—may also inhibit young athletes from seeking help for their problems.

Superior Physical Ability May Mask Health Problems

Athletes who are gifted with extraordinary natural abilities or who are in exceptional physical condition can often develop health problems or engage in risky behavior without demonstrating serious symptoms. Many athletes may be able to use tobacco, alcohol, or other drugs and yet be able to perform at an acceptable level due to superior ability or conditioning. Some athletes are able to conceal their serious problems over a long period of time without a noticeable diminishing of athletic performance. Some coaches may be willing to ignore tobacco, alcohol, or other drug use if it is not affecting the athlete's performance.

Myths About Athletes and Athletics

Some of the long-standing and cherished beliefs about athletics may foster a willingness of a community to turn its head when problems occur. Many people believe that athletes do not use tobacco, alcohol, or other drugs, that athletes are the "good kids," and that other kids are the ones who use drugs. This belief may lead them to focus on students they believe are at higher risk and forget about the needs of athletes.

Immediate Intervention

The previous information in this chapter specified what to do when you are concerned about an athlete in nonemergency situations. In emergency situations involving threat to the health or safety of the athlete or others, an immediate response is necessary. Once an emergency situation is resolved, then the information given previously—about identifying behavior, sharing concern, upholding expectations, and referring and supporting an athlete—still applies. An immediate response is necessary in the following circumstances:

1. Behavior that jeopardizes the athlete's own health or safety. If the situation is a medical emergency, use first-aid procedures (or obtain assistance to apply first aid to the athlete), and contact emergency medical help. If the situation involves overdose or withdrawal, attempt to determine the type of drug taken. In certain emergency circumstances, you may need to initiate a search of clothing or lockers, contact friends and teammates, and carefully observe any odors or behaviors that might indicate the type of drug used.

2. An athlete's behavior threatens the health or safety of a staff member or another student. Take whatever immediate steps you can to secure the area, then contact school security, administration, or local law enforcement.

3. An athlete is observed possessing, selling, or using tobacco, alcohol, or other drugs in violation of state or federal laws. In this case, appropriate authorities will be contacted. Usually, this will be the school administrator's responsibility, but you may need to contact local officials directly in some emergency situations.

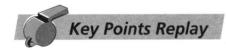

Key Points Replay

■ As a coach, you are in a good position to observe, identify, and respond to your athletes' behavior.

■ The behaviors you observe could be caused by a variety of problems. It is not necessary to know what causes the behavior before you respond. Focus on behavior. Avoid diagnosing the problem or labeling the athlete.

■ Your relationship with your athletes provides an opportunity for you to share your concern, support them, and refer them, if necessary, to someone else.

■ As well as sharing your concern with and supporting an athlete, you need to uphold the expectations you have set for the athlete and the team.

■ Although you may be the best person to notice something is troubling an athlete, you may not be the best person to help resolve the problem. You should have a key contact to provide backup when referring students for additional help.

Part

III

Calling on Reserves

Part III of *Coaches Guide to Drugs and Sport* explores resources available in the school and community to help you respond to troubled athletes and use educational resources. Part III is based on the philosophy that you do not have to take on the job of preventing tobacco, alcohol, and other drug problems or of responding to troubled students by yourself.

As you read the next five chapters, you will find out how an organized, school-based approach, called a student assistance program, can provide systematic and coordinated help for students and their parents. You will explore community resources that are available to help athletes who are experiencing problems with tobacco, alcohol, and other drugs. You will also find guidance in these pages about choosing resources for your educational sessions with athletes and their parents, and you will learn about the advantages and disadvantages of drug testing in the high school.

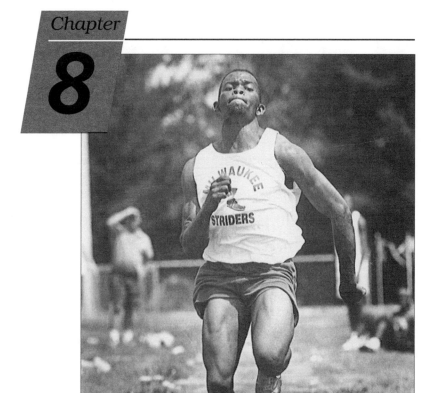

The Student Assistance Approach

Chapter Warm-Up

Chapter 8 will help you understand four approaches to student assistance programs. You will learn how to figure out what approach your school uses and what kinds of services might be available for you, your athletes, and their parents.

What Are Student Assistance Programs?

School-based student assistance programs are built on the philosophy and experience of now well-established employee assistance programs. In the early 1970s, it became evident that alcohol and other drug problems were taking a major toll on business and industry. At the same time, treatment programs were showing promise in rehabilitating employees. Thus, occupational alcoholism programs were born.

They had one major flaw, however: their name. They were known as occupational alcoholism programs, which meant an employee had to admit to a problem with alcohol before seeking help or a supervisor had to diagnose an employee as having a problem with alcohol before referring the employee to the occupational alcoholism counselor. Because the stigma surrounding alcoholism was—and is—such a barrier to seeking help, employees and supervisors were reluctant to address the problem. Referrals in the early days of occupational alcoholism programs were low, which meant that many people did not receive the help they needed.

It also became increasingly apparent that the symptoms of alcoholism resembled the symptoms of other problems: depression, family conflict, economic struggles, or illness. Many companies changed the name of their occupational alcoholism program to employee assistance programs. This usually reflected a philosophical shift. Employees could now visit the employee assistance counselor to receive help for any problem that could potentially affect their work. Supervisors no longer needed to confront employees with their concerns about alcohol or other drug use; they could simply describe the behavior that needed to be altered and suggest employee assistance if the employee needed help to make the changes.

At the same time that businesses were developing occupational alcoholism programs, schools were also struggling to figure out how to respond to increasing numbers of young people who were using tobacco, alcohol, and other drugs. With the realization that adolescents could become dependent on alcohol or other drugs,[1] treatment programs designed specifically for young people began to be developed throughout the country. Attention turned to the schools as a logical place to identify young people who were dependent, to provide structured interventions, and to refer them to an assessment or treatment center.

The early school-based programs were intended to focus only on alcohol and other drug dependency. Schools who used this approach reported the same problems as occupational alcoholism programs in business and industry. When they developed programs that focused on identifying students who have tobacco, alcohol, and other drug

In Toms River, New Jersey, all designated captains of the athletic teams met on a monthly basis to provide support as they dealt with leadership issues. This concept, which became known as the "Captains' Table," eventually spread to the entire South Shore District.

---

[1]*Note*: When we refer to dependency, treatment, or aftercare, we will drop the word "tobacco" from our phrase, "tobacco, alcohol, or other drugs." While we strongly believe that nicotine dependence is as serious as any other drug dependency, at the time of this writing, nicotine dependence is still viewed differently by most segments of the treatment community. Unfortunately, the few options available for treating nicotine dependence are generally smoking-cessation programs offered through school or community agencies.

problems, staff were reluctant to refer students, and self-referrals from students were low. A better approach followed on the heels of the early drug-specific programs. Schools began to develop broadbrush programs that provided help for physical, social, psychological, familial, mental, legal, or academic problems. Students learned that they could get help for any problem that was affecting their lives without labeling themselves or disclosing themselves to more people than they wanted. Staff realized that they did not have to know what the underlying problem was before they could respond. Many programs began to report increased referrals from staff and from students, and the concept of a broadbrush student assistance program became a reality.

What Can I Expect From a Student Assistance Program?

This section will describe four approaches to student assistance now in place throughout the country. Understanding these approaches will help you determine what kind of help you can expect for your athletes from a student assistance program. The approaches differ in both focus and scope.

Some student assistance programs (Table 8.1) limit their focus to tobacco, alcohol, and other drug-use problems. Others take the broadbrush approach described above and respond to all problems that affect young people. Some student assistance programs limit their scope only to intervention. These programs provide a systematic way of responding to student problems and do not provide prevention and health-promotion services. Others take an umbrella approach and provide intervention, prevention, and health-promotion services. (For the purpose of this discussion, we define

Table 8.1 Types of Student Assistance Programs

	Type 1: Problem-specific intervention	Type 2: Problem-specific combination	Type 3: Broadbrush intervention	Type 4: Broadbrush combination
Intervention for students with tobacco, alcohol, and other drug problems	x	x		
Intervention for students who are experiencing any problem.			x	x
Prevention and health promotion to resolve tobacco, alcohol, and other drug problems		x		
Prevention and health promotion to resolve any adolescent problem				x

prevention as "actions taken to reduce the incidence of specific problems, such as tobacco, alcohol, and other drug use." We define health promotion as "actions taken to support and enhance overall health." The approaches are described here from the most limited in focus and scope to the broadest.

Type 1: Problem-Specific Student Assistance Programs (Intervention)

These programs provide a structured approach to identifying and responding to students who are experiencing tobacco, alcohol, and other drug problems. They usually offer counseling and support groups but do not coordinate prevention or health promotion programs. If your school has this type of program, student assistance staff could probably do the following:

- Consult with you when you become concerned about an athlete who might be experiencing tobacco-, alcohol-, and other drug-use problems.
- Gather information to determine if an athlete needs help to resolve tobacco-, alcohol-, and other drug-use problems.
- Refer athletes or their families to appropriate resources within or outside of the school for help with tobacco-, alcohol-, and other drug-use problems.
- Provide follow-up for students and their families.
- Conduct or find a support group to help an athlete resolve tobacco, alcohol, and other drug-use problems.
- Work with an athlete's parents to help the athlete remain abstinent from the use of tobacco, alcohol, or other drugs.
- Share information on tobacco, alcohol, and other drug problems and the services they provide at a preseason meeting.
- Offer staff inservice training for coaches on tobacco, alcohol, and other drugs.

Type 2: Problem-Specific Student Assistance Programs (Health Promotion, Prevention, Intervention)

Like Type 1 programs, these programs focus on tobacco, alcohol, and other drug problems only, but the scope of their services may include prevention and health promotion. If your school has this type of program, student assistance staff will provide the same services described in Type 1, and they may also offer the following services:

- Help you organize and facilitate a preseason meeting and find speakers, audiovisual materials, and other resources to provide information on tobacco-, alcohol-, and other drug-use issues.
- Put you in contact with parent groups who could organize alternative activities for your team.
- Locate or arrange leadership training opportunities to support drug-free team leaders.

- Provide educational sessions for your team on tobacco, alcohol, and other drugs.
- Offer staff inservice training for coaches on prevention and health promotion topics related to tobacco, alcohol, and other drugs.

Type 3: Broadbrush Student Assistance Programs (Intervention)

Like Type 1 programs, these programs limit their scope to identifying and responding to troubled students. However, they have a broader focus, encouraging referrals for any problem affecting students. If your school has this type of program, student assistance staff could probably provide the following services, which are parallel to the services described for the Type 1 program, but are broader in focus:

- Consult with you when you become concerned—for any reason—about an athlete.
- Gather information to determine if an athlete needs help to resolve a personal issue.
- Refer athletes or their families to appropriate resources within or outside of the school for help.
- Provide case management and follow-up for students and their families.
- Conduct or find a support group to help an athlete resolve personal problems or maintain a healthy lifestyle.
- Work with an athlete's parents to help the athlete achieve personal goals.
- Share information at a preseason meeting about problems that affect young people and the services they provide.
- Offer staff inservice training for coaches on how to refer to and work with the student assistance program.

Type 4: Broadbrush Student Assistance Programs (Health Promotion, Prevention, Intervention)

These programs are the broadest in both focus and scope. They offer a one-stop shop for all student needs—including academic concerns—often acting as an umbrella for all student services. Their scope may include prevention, health promotion, and intervention with a broad focus on all types of problems that affect students. If your school has this type of program, student assistance staff could provide all of the services described in the Type 3 programs, as well as the following:

- Help you organize a preseason meeting and find speakers, audiovisual materials, and other resources to provide information on a variety of healthy-lifestyle issues;
- Put you in contact with parent groups who could organize alternative activities for your team;
- Locate or arrange leadership training for your team leaders;

- Provide educational sessions for your team on a variety of healthy-lifestyle issues; and

- Provide staff inservice training for coaches on a variety of health-related issues, covering prevention, health promotion, and intervention topics.

How Do I Find Out What Type of Program Our School Has?

In our experience, the best way to find out about your school's student assistance program is to meet with your school's student assistance coordinator or student assistance counselor. Request a copy of any policies and procedures that govern the functioning of the student assistance program and ask questions like the following:

- What is the focus of the program? What problems does the student assistance program address? Just tobacco, alcohol, and other drugs, or any problem affecting young people?

- What is the scope of the program? What services does it offer? In addition to assessment and referral, what other services does the program provide? These services could include prevention or health promotion education, leadership training, staff training, teacher-coach consultation, counseling, and support groups.

- As a coach, how do I use these services? How will these services benefit my athletes and their parents?

- Who is directly involved in the student assistance program? Is there a team? How often do they meet? How are staff, students, and parents involved?

- If I need to make a referral, to whom would it go? What forms need to be completed? What can I expect to hear about the referral, and how soon can I expect to hear?

- How can I support the student assistance program? Options may include: being a member of the student assistance team, spreading the word about the student assistance program to team members and their parents, talking to colleagues about the student assistance program, and attending educational sessions if they are offered.

What If My School Does Not Have a Student Assistance Program?

While we believe strongly in its benefits, many schools do not have a student assistance program available for students and staff. The size of the school or the staffing pattern may simply not warrant this approach, a school may be philosophically opposed to providing assistance to students for personal problems, or it may prefer other approaches. As a coach, you still need backup in order to respond appropriately to athletes who are experiencing problems. Chapter 7 discussed the importance of identifying a key contact who can provide assistance to students once you have done everything you can do as a coach. If your school does not have a key contact through a structured student assistance program as described in this chapter, you can still find a key contact in the school or in the community who can help. This key contact may be an individual counselor, social worker, psychologist, nurse, or administrator. Whoever your key contact is, that person should be knowledgeable about school and community resources for adolescents, be able to work with young people and their families to find the right sources of help, and be connected appropriately to the school in order to provide confidential services for students. See "Referring" for a list of other helpful characteristics in a key contact (p. 87-88)

Another option is to a help implement a student assistance program in your school. The next chapter will discuss the team approach to student assistance and let you know what you, as a coach, can expect from this type of student assistance program. It will also give you some suggestions for starting a student assistance program if your school does not already have one.

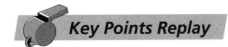

Key Points Replay

- Student assistance programs may vary in both focus and scope and differ from school to school, based on the philosophy of the school and community.

- The focus of a student assistance program may be either problem-specific, focusing only on tobacco, alcohol, or other drugs, or broadbrush, focusing on all problems that may affect adolescents.

- The scope of a student assistance program may be either limited to intervention (identifying and responding to troubled students) or include prevention and health promotion activities.

- As a coach, you can find out about your school's student assistance program by meeting with its coordinator, asking appropriate questions, and requesting copies of policies and procedures.

- If your school does not have a student assistance program, you can still find a key contact in the school or community who can back you up when you are concerned about one of your athletes.

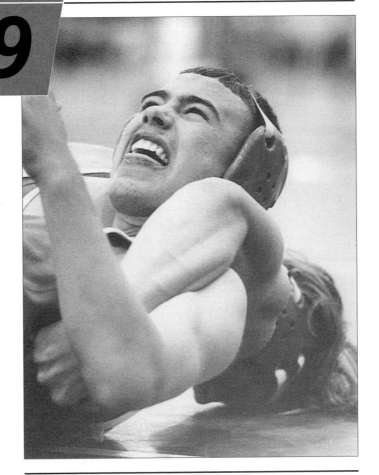

Responding to Students' Needs

Chapter Warm-Up

Chapter 9 will help you interact more effectively with your school's student assistance program. You will learn about the advantages of the team approach to student assistance and understand what happens once you have referred a student to the program for help.

Chapter 8 described four approaches to student assistance. Regardless of the type of student assistance program your school has in place, all should be able to provide assistance to your athletes who are experiencing problems with tobacco, alcohol, and other drugs. We believe that student assistance programs that have a broad focus offer distinct advantages over problem-specific approaches:

- One referral form and one referral process can be developed for all student concerns.
- This one-stop shop reduces confusion on the part of staff because they do not have to figure out either what the underlying problem is or to whom they should refer a student.
- The need for specialized, inservice training for staff on child abuse; tobacco, alcohol, and other drug use; special education; sexual abuse; and other issues is reduced.
- Coaching and teaching staff feel supported in their efforts, and they are freed of the need to be experts in all of these areas or to provide counseling for students.
- Students are given help in a more systematic and consistent way.
- Communication is increased between educational and support staff.

However, having made a case for a broadbrush student assistance program, we recognize that both the focus and the scope of the program may differ depending on the philosophy and resources of the school. Because *Coaches Guide to Drugs and Sport* limits its focus to tobacco, alcohol, and other drugs, the next part of the chapter will concentrate on the role of a student assistance program in responding to athletes who are experiencing problems in this area of their lives.

The Team Approach to Student Assistance

We highly recommend that a team of people be pulled together to address the needs of students. This approach reduces the fragmentation and duplication of effort that naturally occurs without such a team. A student assistance team is made up of representatives from all areas of the academic, cocurricular, and support services within the school. Usually, the team includes anyone who has a designated responsibility for providing special services for students: administrators, guidance counselors, school nurses, social workers, school psychologists, special education staff, and coordinators of special programs (such as a coordinator of programs for gifted students or a prevention specialist). Ideally, it also includes a representative from the cocurricular area, such as an athletic director. Some schools also include academic staff on a half-time or rotating basis. It should not include students or parents because of the need to maintain confidentiality. Following are some of the advantages of a student assistance team.

Better Understanding of the Students' Needs

Different team members bring together diverse sets of information, experience, skills, and approaches. This allows the team to get a better understanding of a student's needs in order to provide a more thorough assessment. For instance, a school nurse may look more closely at the health needs of a student, while a school social worker may be more sensitive to the student's family needs. If these professionals are working in isolation, they may tend to see only one perspective, as in the old adage, "If the only tool you have is a hammer, everything looks like a nail."

More Productive Use of Time

Regular team meetings reduce time spent coordinating schedules between team members who would have to connect with each other anyway. For instance, a school counselor may need to obtain information from a school administrator who would need to meet with an attendance officer. If they regularly meet on Wednesday mornings, they may not need to spend time exchanging phone messages or comparing daily schedules.

Better Distribution of Workload

In the team approach, the responsibilities for data collection and case management are distributed more equally throughout the team.

Improved Communication With Staff

A team approach to student assistance allows more coordinated and effective communication with staff. Without a team approach, for instance, a third-hour teacher might be contacted by the school principal, the school psychologist, and the guidance counselor about the same student for the same problem.

Less Confusion About Referral Procedures

When staff know that the student assistance team handles any type of student concern, they do not have to figure out which staff member is most appropriate to help them each time they have a concern about a student.

Better Follow-Up for Students and Staff

The regularity of team meetings coupled with a structured process for follow-up can reduce the chance that a student will fall through the cracks. Student assistance programs have built-in accountability.

What Does a Student Assistance Team Do?

Chapter 7 covered information about identifying behaviors of concern, talking to an athlete about your concerns, and referring when necessary. This chapter and chapter 10 will take you through the next steps of the process (Figure 9.1).

Assistance Process

Staff member

Athletic director or
coach

Observes and identifies
behavior
Shares concern
Upholds expectations
Provides support
Refers, if appropriate

Key contact

Student assistance team
or key contact

ACCEPTS REFERRALS
**COMMUNICATES WITH YOUNG
PERSON, OTHER STAFF, AND
PARENTS**
GATHERS INFORMATION
MAKES A PRE-ASSESSMENT
SETS GOALS AND DEVELOPS A PLAN
PROVIDES SUPPORT
**REFERS TO ADDITIONAL
RESOURCES, IF APPROPRIATE**

**School or community
resource**

Continues assessment
Provides education,
counseling, and treatment
Offers aftercare and other
support

Figure 9.1   Assistance process emphasizing chapter 9 stages.
Adapted from Harding, Ringhofer & Associates, Inc., 1994.

Accepts Referrals

The student assistance team is responsible for handling all referrals from staff, students, and parents. They will usually develop a referral form which will ask you to provide information that can help them determine what specific problems the young person is experiencing. At a minimum, the form will ask you to record the date and time of any significant incident(s), the location (for example, in the classroom, in the hallway, or in the locker room), and a description of the behavior and any actions you have already taken (e.g., you have talked to the student, notified parents, or benched or suspended the athlete for a period of time). The form may include a checklist of possible student behaviors. If it does not, remember to be specific about the behaviors in order to reduce misunderstanding (Figure 9.2).

The following case study will illustrate this process from the time a coach made a referral to the student assistance team. This situation is fictitious and represents the ideal of how student assistance teams can function. We recognize that not all situations are resolved so satisfactorily.

Jason Brown is a senior in high school and plays basketball on your varsity team. He is a good student with a current 3.4 GPA. As his coach, you are pleased to have him on your team because he is a good team player, responsible, and dedicated. Recently, however, you have become concerned about Jason. He has been showing up a little late for practice, his energy level during drills is low, and on Tuesday he got in a loud argument with a teammate, stomped off the court, and left practice without talking to anybody. When you talked to Jason on Wednesday, he said that he just had a lot on his mind with finals coming up and that he would be fine and you should not be concerned. You reminded him about your expectations regarding attendance and treating teammates with respect. On Thursday, however, Jason skipped practice. You talked with one of his teammates who said that he was concerned about Jason, too, but did not want to "rat on him." Today (Friday) you caught Jason in the hall between classes and told him that you would like to talk to him. He refused to talk, simply looking at the floor as you spoke. You told him you were concerned about him, that you wanted to keep him on the team, and that you were going to ask someone from the student assistance team to talk to him because he did not want to talk to you. He said, "Fine, coach, you can do what you want, but I don't have to talk to them." You reminded Jason of the expectations you had about attending practice and told him that because he skipped practice yesterday, he could not play in tonight's game. You also asked him to suit up and be on the bench. After he left your office, you filled out a referral.

Most student assistance teams meet on a regular basis (every week or every two weeks, depending on the size of the school building). At each meeting, they review any referrals they have received and divide the referrals among the members of the team. These "case managers" do their homework before the next team meeting in order to get as clear a picture as possible about what is happening in the young person's life that resulted in the referral. They will be responsible for following and supporting this student—and the student's

The _____ [name of school] student assistance program is intended to systematically and professionally respond to the problems of students. This request-for-assistance form is intended to provide school staff an opportunity to involve a student demonstrating problematic behavior with our student assistance program pre-assessment team so that his/her problem might be resolved.

Please complete this form as accurately and thoroughly as you can. The information you provide may be shared with the student and his/her parents at the professional discretion of the student assistance program pre-assessment team.

Thank you for your cooperation and concern.

List specific student behavior that seems problematic to you. Be as specific as possible.

Behavior	Location	Time & date

List specific actions that you have taken in response to these behaviors.

Your action	Location	Time & date	Student's response to your action

Thank you for your referral of _____, _____, to the pre-assessment team. The
(Student's name)   (Date)

pre-assessment team will be taking appropriate action.

Figure 9.2   Example of a request-for-assistance form.

Reprinted from Funk, Svendsen, Cunningham, and Griffin (1989).

family, when appropriate—through the process, helping to remove any roadblocks that arise.

On Monday morning one of the student assistance team members is stopped in the hallway by an 11th grader who asks to talk. He says he is concerned about one of his basketball teammates who was at a party on Friday night. He says the teammate was drunk, and he does not know what to do about it. He has seen this teammate do this before, and it is really bothering him because the team has made a nonuse pledge for the season. He has thought about telling the coach, but he does not know if the coach will do anything about it. Besides, his teammate was already benched on Friday night for skipping practice. If the coach does suspend the teammate, he's afraid the other players will think he was the one who told the coach. He is coming to the student assistance team because he heard the team could keep things confidential. He is willing to give the teammate's name and fill out a referral form, but he wants to remain anonymous. He tells the student assistance team member that the player's name is Jason Brown. When the members of the student assistance team meet for their regular Monday-afternoon session, they have your referral and the teammate's referral on Jason Brown. The team decides that action needs to be taken quickly and asks Ms. Edwards to be the case manager for Jason because she has a good relationship with him and his friends. Ms. Edwards is the high school social studies teacher who is serving a one-year appointment on the student assistance team as the faculty representative.

Communicates With Young Person, Other Staff, and Parents

The case manager may call you to get more information about the referral you made. In addition, the case manager may talk to other school staff and, if appropriate, to students' parents. In most instances, the case manager will interview the young person to get the athlete's perceptions.

Ms. Edwards calls you to thank you for referring Jason, to let you know that the referral seems appropriate, and that she will be talking to Jason soon. She asks you if you have any more information you would like to share and particularly if you have any concerns about Jason's use of tobacco, alcohol, or other drugs. You tell her that, although you would not be surprised if Jason was drinking (because lots of high school students do), you do not have any particular reason to suspect him of using.

Ms. Edwards also talks to another teammate, the English teacher, and to Jason. Rather reluctantly, the teammate tells Ms. Edwards that he is concerned about Jason's drinking because the amount he is drinking seems to be increasing. However, the teammate says that even though Jason never seems to be drunk, he is concerned about him, particularly when Jason drives. Jason's English teacher says that he did poorly on his English final and has been performing erratically in class; sometimes he skips class and says that he does not feel well. The English teacher has noticed an increasing concern on Jason's part about basketball and getting a college scholarship. When Ms. Edwards talks to Jason, he denies using any drugs other than alcohol. He admits to occasional alcohol use in the past but denies any recent use because of the basketball team's policy and pledge of nonuse. He denies use at any specific times or situations. He asks how Ms. Edwards got his information and starts guessing about who might have told on him.

Gathers Information

The case manager will also obtain school records on grades, school attendance (including both absences and tardiness), and participation in cocurricular activities. In some cases, the case manager may also obtain information outside the school from other institutions, such as court services or social services.

> Ms. Edwards talks to the school secretary, who checks attendance and finds out that Jason has missed an average amount of school this school year—about the same amount he missed last year. However, recent absences have been unexcused. The secretary also checks his grades and finds that, although they have dropped in the past term, they are still above average.

Makes a Pre-Assessment

Throughout this process, the case manager will attempt to get a clear picture of the student and the student's problems in order to determine if the reported concern is either an isolated incident or part of a larger pattern. The case manager will also begin to determine the strengths and limitations of the student, potential barriers to resolving the problem behavior, and the level of support available to the student. By the end of this information-gathering period, the case manager may be able to identify what the major issues are for the student, or may ask the team for assistance in identifying these issues. It is important to note that this pre-assessment is different than a medical or psychological diagnosis. It is simply a decision about whether the problem behavior can be appropriately addressed within the educational setting or whether the student and the parents should be referred to an outside resource. It is an educated guess—based on available data—about which areas should be further explored by professionals either within or outside the school setting.

> By this time, Ms. Edwards has only a sketchy picture of Jason's situation. She knows that you, as his coach, have concerns about his performance. She knows that Jason's teammate is concerned about his alcohol use, and she knows that Jason's grades are satisfactory but at least one of his teachers is concerned. She also knows that Jason's attendance is not as good as it should be. Ms. Edwards asks the team for help; the consensus is that it would be appropriate for Ms. Edwards, the school counselor, Jason, and Jason's parents to meet for a conference.

Sets Goals and Develops a Plan

Once the team has come to an agreement about the student's primary needs, they will assist the case manager in setting goals and developing a plan for the student. This plan may include referral to an outside agency for further assessment or treatment or a referral to resources within the school setting that can help the student. Or the team may decide that no further action is necessary at this time. The plan would then simply be to document the incident that led to the referral and communicate with the person who referred.

In this case, the student assistance team's plan was simply to get more information. Ms. Edwards followed the advice of the team and scheduled a conference with Jason, the school counselor, and Jason's father. Mr. Brown was very proud of Jason's accomplishments. He had encouraged Jason in his activities and was especially proud of how he performed in basketball. Jason's chances for a college scholarship delighted Mr. Brown because he was not sure how he could pay for a college education. He passed off Ms. Edward's concerns about Jason as "senioritis" and said that he was sure that Jason did not drink alcohol. Mr. Brown said he would come in for a conference, although he did not think it was at all necessary for a student who was getting good grades, anyway. When the conference was held, Jason held fast to his contention that he had no problems and that he could just do what everybody wanted: come to class, go to practice, get good grades, and live up to everybody's "stupid" expectations. When the conference was over, however, Jason's father confided to the school counselor that he had found beer cans in the back of his truck last Friday night and that he and Jason were not getting along right now. He asked the counselor not to tell the coach, because he was afraid Jason would get kicked off the team.

Provides Support

Once this plan has been developed, the case manager will meet with the student and the parents (when appropriate) to talk about the plan and offer support. At this point, the plan may be revised or refined, based on the needs and wishes of the student and the family. These changes would be reported back to the team.

The school counselor suggested to Jason's father that he take Jason to the Riverside Adolescent Center for an assessment. The school counselor said that Jason's reluctance to talk about the situation at school, coupled with serious concerns from his father and from his teammate, suggested that someone other than the school should find out the degree of Jason's problems with alcohol or other drugs. Jason's father said that he would think about it and talk to Jason. Two days later, Jason's father called the school counselor and asked for more information about the assessment center. Ms. Edwards reported this information back to the student assistance team, who suggested that Ms. Edwards call Jason's father back in a week to follow up.

Refers to Additional Resources

The plan may include referral to an agency outside of the school for further assessment (such as a mental health agency or a treatment center) or to an internal resource (such as a special education program, a guidance counselor, or a support group). If appropriate, the case manager may help the student and the family make the appointment and follow up to see if the family needs further assistance.

Ms. Edwards called Jason's father in one week, but no one answered the phone. She left messages at home and at Mr. Brown's workplace, but they were not returned. When Ms. Edwards talked to Jason, he said, "Oh, that. Yeah, Dad made some noise about going somewhere, but we didn't."

Provides Follow-Up

The case manager will also contact you—as the person who referred the student—to let you know what has happened. Because of confidentiality restrictions, the case manager may only be able to give you limited information. At the very least, you have the right to know that the assistance team has met to consider your referral.

Ms. Edwards called you and, once again, thanked you for your referral, told you it was appropriate, and asked you to stay in touch with the student assistance team and to let them know if anything changed. She thanked you for your concern about Jason and for taking action. When you asked for more information, she told you that confidentiality required her not to disclose anything more. You were frustrated because Jason's performance was just adequate. You knew he could do better.

The student assistance team's job with the student continues until the behavior that resulted in the referral changes. If the behavior does not change, the process will be reactivated. Often the student assistance team will set a reasonable time for changes to occur and will then check back with you to see either if things have been resolved or if you still have concerns about your athlete.

The student assistance team had set a standard time of 60 days to check to see how Jason was doing. However, in less than a month, Jason's father was back in the counselor's office. Jason had taken his father's car without permission and had not come home when expected. Mr. Brown was worried and had been up all night. When Jason finally came home at 5:00 a.m., he smelled like alcohol. The car was dented on the front fender. Although Jason had not been picked up by the police, Mr. Brown was sure Jason had been driving after he was drinking. He was furious at Jason and was worried about him. He asked for the school counselor's help in getting Jason to the assessment office. The school counselor gave him the name of his key contact at the Riverside Assessment Center and offered to help him make the appointment. Mr. Brown left the office and, this time, followed through by keeping the appointment that the school counselor made.

Once I Make a Referral, How Do I Support an Athlete?

As a coach, you may be one of the most important influences in a young person's life. A referral to a student assistance program can be extremely threatening to a young person if they feel that this referral severs your relationship. You play a key role in the student assistance process by providing ongoing support for your athletes. This section will give you some ideas about ways you might be able to provide this support.

Support at the Time of Referral

Chapter 7 discussed ways to respond appropriately when you are concerned about an athlete. When it is necessary to refer an athlete to someone else for help, the most important thing you can do during this process is to let the young person know that you are making the referral because you care and because you think the referral is in the athlete's best interest. Only rarely will you make a referral without the athlete's knowledge. When you talk with the athlete, the athlete may tell you about a personal or family concern which is obviously beyond your ability to help. In this case, you will probably discuss the necessity of seeking help and offer to go with the athlete to see the student assistance counselor. The student may refuse to talk about the situation, react belligerently, and refuse to change. You may need to refer the student to the student assistance program in order to help resolve the situation. Usually, you will tell the student that if the behavior does not change, you will need to make a referral. You may still offer to go with the student to see the student assistance counselor, but if the student is upset about your discussion, your offer may be refused.

Support During the Pre-Assessment Process

During the time the student assistance team is meeting, your support is best offered through your natural relationship to the athlete as that person's coach. You may simply be available to talk with the athlete and ask how things are going—without prying. Be alert to cues about what the athlete may need from you. Remember that once you have referred an athlete to the student assistance program, what happens next is strictly confidential. You may never know what the actual problem is with your athlete or the outcome of the referral. Although this may seem frustrating, it is essential that athletes know that what they share with a student assistance counselor or a student assistance team member will be kept private. Otherwise, the entire program is in jeopardy. Data privacy laws also govern the amount and types of information that can be shared.

Support During Treatment

In certain circumstances, however, you may know that an athlete has been referred to a treatment program outside of the school. This information may come from the athlete, the family, or from a counselor if the athlete or the family has given permission for this information to be shared with you. In this privileged instance, you may choose to play a more important role during treatment. If an athlete is involved in inpatient treatment, you may certainly offer the same kind of support you would if an athlete was involved in any other type of hospitalization: cards, flowers, or perhaps visits to the treatment center. You may have such a close relationship with the athlete that the athlete may ask for you to be involved during the treatment process by attending an educational or counseling session.

Support Following Treatment

Adolescents who go through treatment for alcohol or other drug dependency often have a very tough time once they return to the school environment. Their friends usually are their drinking or using buddies. So, evenings, weekends, and lunch hours can be difficult and risky times if the student cannot establish friendships with young people who are nonusers. Treatment programs often recommend that young people establish entirely new friendship groups, but this is not easy. Social groups in schools are usually well-defined, with little movement among them. Nonusers may be skeptical of a peer's commitment to nonuse and unwilling to admit someone with a heavy drinking or using history to their group. An athlete's using group of friends may be very willing to welcome that athlete back but not supportive of the choice to not use. Even if these friends are supportive of the athlete's choice not to use, they will probably continue to go to the same drinking parties or gather where other drugs are around. The student may simply not be ready to change groups because that student may not see the need to find new friends. In any case, this is where your role comes in: You can help the young person find a new group of friends and help the athlete to handle situations where an old group of friends is advocating use. You can offer this support in several ways:

- Introduce the student to a group of athletes who have chosen not to use tobacco, alcohol, and other drugs, and who may be involved in prevention efforts.
- Talk to the team—with the athlete's permission, of course—about involvement in treatment and goals for recovery. You may also encourage some athletes to talk to the team themselves.
- Encourage the athlete to follow through with the treatment recommendations, for example, attending in-school support groups, AA, or NA groups (see chapter 10 for more information on these programs).
- Ask parents and student athletes to organize aftergame events or activities that provide a drug-free environment at high-risk times.
- Continue to use the strategies presented earlier in *Coaches Guide to Drugs and Sport* that promote the nonuse of tobacco, alcohol, and other drugs.
- Treat the athlete just as you would any of the other athletes you coach: provide encouragement, teach skills, and recognize accomplishment. Involvement in a cocurricular activity under your direction can provide a healthy, structured environment that can

help a young athlete remain free of tobacco, alcohol, and other drug use.

- Do not give up on the athlete. Recovery is difficult for young people, and many will relapse. According to your athletic policy, it may not be possible for some young people to remain on your team. However, you can still stay in contact and, in so doing, send a clear message that the athlete is important to you as a person, not just as an athlete.

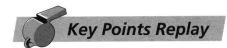

Key Points Replay

■ When a student assistance program focuses on a wide range of problems affecting young people, staff, students, and parents do not have to diagnose a problem in order to access services.

■ When a school uses a team approach to student assistance, services can be provided more systematically and thoroughly than when individual staff act in isolation to help students.

■ The function of a student assistance team is to communicate with the young person, other staff, and parents (if appropriate); gather information; make a pre-assessment; set goals and develop a plan; provide support; refer to additional resources; and provide follow-up.

■ As a coach, there are many ways you can support athletes as they go through the student assistance process.

10

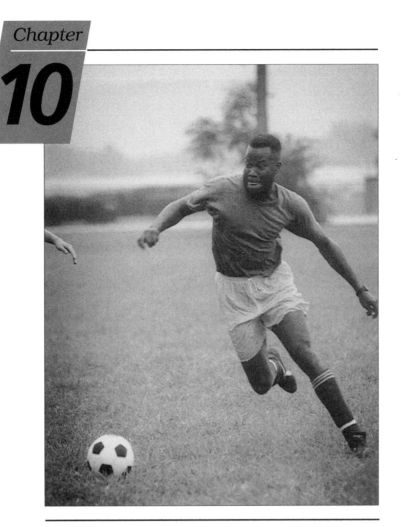

Finding Help in the School and Community

Chapter 10 will help you identify a wide range of resources that are available in the school and community to help young people who are experiencing problems with tobacco, alcohol, and other drugs. Although it is not your job to keep track of these resources, knowing about them will help you support your athletes as they use these resources. If your school does not have a student assistance program, you will learn how you can be a catalyst for getting one started.

Chapter 9 described a team approach to student assistance and gave an overview of what happens once a student is referred to a student assistance program. If the student assistance team determines through this process that the young person needs further help to resolve personal problems, the team will make a referral to either a school or a community resource. This chapter will describe the four roles that a school or community resource can play: assessment; education; counseling and treatment; and aftercare or other support. Figure 10.1 shows the areas of the assistance-process flowchart that this chapter will cover.

Assistance Process

Staff member

Athletic director or
coach

Observes and identifies
  behavior
Shares concern
Upholds expectations
Provides support
Refers, if appropriate

Key contact

Student assistance team
or key contact

Accepts referrals
Communicates with young person,
  other staff, and parents
Gathers information
Makes a pre-assessment
Sets goals and develops a plan
Provides support
Refers to additional resources,
  if appropriate

School or community
resource

CONTINUES ASSESSMENT
PROVIDES EDUCATION,
  COUNSELING, AND
  TREATMENT
OFFERS AFTERCARE AND
  OTHER SUPPORT

Figure 10.1   Assistance process emphasizing chapter 10 stages.
Adapted from Harding, Ringhofer & Associates, Inc., 1994.

Assessment and Evaluation

First we will look at the resources that may be available in a school or community for helping to determine what course of action is appropriate for students.

School-Based Assessment

As described in chapter 9, the student assistance team communicates with staff, students, and parents, gathers information from school records, and discusses this information at a team meeting. Through this process, the team may decide that a more thorough assessment, which may include an assessment of tobacco, alcohol, and other drug use, would be helpful. Many schools have social workers, psychologists, or counselors available who can conduct a more intensive adolescent assessment, including a determination of the young person's relationship to tobacco, alcohol, and other drugs. Often these professionals have had special training in intervention or counseling in the area of tobacco-, alcohol-, and other drug-use problems. It must be noted, however, that their assessment still does not constitute a diagnostic evaluation for dependency. It is simply a more thorough examination of the student's tobacco, alcohol, and other drug use and may eventually result in a referral to an outside agency for further evaluation. The school professional who conducts the assessment will refer to school-based resources if the professional determines that the student is probably not dependent on tobacco, alcohol, or other drugs and that the school has resources that can assist the student. For example, a student may have family problems that stem from the use of tobacco, alcohol, and other drugs, and the school has a student group for students who are coping with a family member's use.

> In Jason Brown's case (chapter 9), the student assistance team determined that Jason was not willing—for whatever reason—to discuss his tobacco, alcohol, or other drug use with school personnel. They therefore suggested to his father that Jason see an assessment specialist in the community. After an incident during which Jason's drinking and driving prompted his father to seek help, they participated in the Riverside Outpatient Treatment Program.

Community-Based Assessment and Evaluation

The student assistance team's assessment responsibility is primarily to determine if a student's needs can be met within the school setting. If not, then the school will refer the student and the parents to an outside school setting where they can obtain an evaluation and diagnostic services. It is often not easy to determine whether an adolescent is dependent on the use of tobacco, alcohol, or other drugs. As with any illness in its early stages, the symptoms may resemble other problems. In addition, young people have usually not established a long history of use, have often not become physically dependent on the drug, and may not have experienced repeated negative consequences. As with adults, the primary indicator of dependency is loss of control, and it is this loss of control over drug use that evaluators will be examining. When a person starts heavy use as an adolescent, dependency may take less time to develop than when a person starts heavy use as an adult. A person does not need to be physically addicted to a drug in order to be dependent on its use.

> The counselors at the assessment agency conducted a thorough assessment of Jason's use of tobacco, alcohol, and other drugs. For Jason, his use had progressed to the point that he was drinking alcohol daily, although usually off school premises. He was drinking heavily on weekends and during the summer. He cut back on his drinking during basketball season but still used. Although he occasionally used marijuana and other drugs if they were available, he preferred to drink alcohol. Jason associated both with teammates who used alcohol and with those who did not, although most of his friends were drinkers. Jason felt that alcohol had become a big part of his life. Despite several attempts to stop using—particularly during the basketball season—Jason relapsed into drinking, usually while attending parties.

Information and Education on Tobacco, Alcohol, and Other Drugs

Based on the data that is available at the time of assessment, staff may determine that a young person is not—at the present time—dependent on the use of tobacco, alcohol, or other drugs. This usually means that staff cannot substantiate that the young person has lost control of use. Still, there was a pattern of use or other inappropriate behavior that initially resulted in the referral. In this case, the staff may refer the athlete to a program that provides education about tobacco, alcohol, and other drug use and teaches skills that the young person needs to change behavior. Once again, these may be school- or community-based.

School-Based Educational Programs

The school may offer educational classes for students who use tobacco, alcohol, and other drugs. These sessions are designed to give information about drug use and teach skills for resisting the pressure to use. They help students examine the importance of tobacco, alcohol, and other drug use in their lives and provide encouragement and support for choosing not to use. Often, these classes are offered as an alternative or addition to a different consequence or penalty. An athlete who has violated a policy for the first time might be appropriate for educational sessions if the student assistance team has determined that there is no evident pattern of alcohol or other drug dependency. These educational sessions may include 2 to 4 meetings and are offered during or after school hours.

Community-Based Educational Programs

Community-based educational programs have similar goals as school-based programs, but may run for a longer period of time. These sessions usually require a parent to attend at least one session. They are often held in the evenings or after school, once or twice a week, for a period of several weeks.

> The assessment counselors at the Riverside Outpatient Treatment Program felt that information and education alone would not help Jason. His many attempts to stop using without success indicated that he needed more intensive help to stop. Jason and his father agreed.

Counseling or Treatment

Professional treatment for alcohol or other drug dependency requires facilities that have skilled professionals available to handle the physical, psychological, emotional, social, and spiritual needs of chemically dependent adolescents and their families.

School-Based Counseling

It is not the school's job to offer treatment for alcohol or other drug dependency. The school may, however, offer short-term, individual counseling in order to help a student and the family establish personal goals and resolve immediate crises. However, for a variety of reasons, group counseling is generally preferable with adolescents, and, therefore, individual counseling is generally seen either as a bridge to support groups within the school or as a stepping-stone to community-based treatment programs.

Community-Based Treatment Options

Community-based treatment options are chosen based on the age of the students, their level of maturity, and how much social support they have.

Outpatient Treatment

Based on the data that is available at the time of assessment, professional staff may determine that a young person is, in fact, dependent on the use of alcohol or other drugs. This means that the young person has lost control of the use and needs more intensive help and support to stop using. The staff will have also assessed the student's level of social support and determined that the family, friends, and school environment would be adequate to support the student's ongoing attendance at outpatient sessions. Outpatient treatment for adolescents may include concurrent sessions with parents. Outpatient treatment sessions are often held in the evenings or after school, four to five times a week, for a period of several weeks. Some communities also offer day treatment for adolescents; such treatment usually includes school attendance and, if necessary, tutoring for part of the day.

> Jason seemed to be an appropriate candidate for outpatient treatment. It appeared that he had a fairly strong level of social support: a father who was willing to back him up, some friends who do not use alcohol, a supportive coach, and support at school. Unfortunately, there were no outpatient treatment programs that were affordable, and Jason's father did not have insurance that would cover the cost of outpatient treatment for adolescents. After much discussion with Jason and his father, the assessment counselors decided to recommend that Jason attend a young person's AA group and suggested that he get involved with his school's abstinence support group at the same time. They facilitated a signed contract between Jason and his father. The contract stipulated that if this approach was not successful—if Jason used again—they would seek inpatient treatment.

Inpatient Treatment

Professional staff may determine that a young person who is dependent on the use of alcohol or other drugs would be unable to function well in an outpatient environment. This decision may be based on the student's need to physically detoxify from alcohol and other drugs, which requires inpatient hospitalization. Outpatient treatment also requires a fairly high level of developmental competency and social support (through family, friends, and school) to be effective. Inpatient treatment provides more structure and intensity, which some adolescents need. Inpatient treatment for adolescents almost always includes a strong family component; family or friends often attend several educational or counseling sessions. Inpatient treatment for adolescents is typically about 4 weeks in duration. Extended care, which can last up to 6 additional months, is sometimes recommended.

Combination of Inpatient and Outpatient Care

Sometimes a combination of approaches will be used. Young people will attend an inpatient program for 1 or 2 weeks and then attend an outpatient program for a few weeks. Insurance coverage often dictates what type of program will be selected and how long the young person will be allowed to participate.

Aftercare and Other Support

Especially for adolescents, support is an essential component of any treatment program. This support can be provided by school- or community-based programs.

School-Based Support Groups

Adolescents spend much of their time at school and with their friends. Thus, school-based support is extremely beneficial in helping young people apply the skills they have learned during treatment to their real, day-to-day lives. They also can form new, supportive friendships when they participate in groups during school. The types of support groups offered by student assistance programs can vary greatly depending on the focus of the program. The type of support group a student assistance program provides should be consistent with the mission and goals of the program. If the program deals primarily with tobacco, alcohol, and other drug use, then the support groups offered should also deal primarily with these issues. If the program has a broad focus, then support groups dealing with other adolescent issues may be offered through the student assistance program.

Problem-Specific Support Groups

These groups provide support for young people who are choosing to change a particular behavior or resolve a specific issue in their lives. Examples of problem-specific approaches for addressing tobacco, alcohol, and other drug problems are aftercare groups for recovering adolescents, support groups for young people who have used before and want to stop, and support groups for adolescents who are living in a home where alcohol and other drugs are a problem.

We have already discussed prevention groups that have a mission to prevent tobacco, alcohol, and other drug problems (chapter 6). These groups often provide alternative activities for students or conduct cross-age or peer education. Although they are not, strictly speaking, support groups, students who attend these groups do obtain a great deal of support for the choices they make to not use tobacco, alcohol, and other drugs. These groups are a natural link between young people who have chosen not to use and those who are recovering from dependency and need to make the same choice each day.

Aftercare Groups.   Young people who return to the school environment following inpatient treatment have special needs for aftercare. Depending on their school environment, their parents, and their friends, they may feel constantly under surveillance or nearly abandoned. Coming back to school, they are faced with the difficulty of needing to establish a new network of friends who do not use. In addition, they must find new activities and interests. Support groups, under the guidance of trained facilitators, can encourage the student to find new friends, to practice skills for avoiding or handling risky situations, to learn new means of handling stress and feeling good without using, and to identify and make progress toward long-term goals.

Family Support Groups.   It is widely recognized that young people who live in homes where parents or siblings are dependent on alcohol or other drugs have special needs. In order to cope with living in these homes, children often learn three rules: do not trust, do not talk, and do not feel. As a result, they often grow up in isolation and feel that no one else has the same problems that they have. They are also at higher risk for their own problems with tobacco, alcohol, and other drug use, and, possibly, other risky behaviors. Schools, recognizing these issues, often offer support groups for students who live in homes where alcohol and other drugs are a problem. Sometimes these groups are called Children of Alcoholics (COA) groups, but we feel that this term could have negative—even legal—implications for a school district. When a student attends a school-sponsored COA group, that student may be admitting to the school that the parents have a problem with alcohol or other drugs. Some schools have avoided this problem by simply providing family support groups or providing unlabeled, general support groups.

Unlabeled, General Support Groups

These groups are provided for adolescents who need support for resolving any issue in their lives. Because they are unlabeled, they do not require the adolescents to diagnose themselves before joining the group, and the groups provide some measure of initial anonymity. When a school has a small student body, these groups also provide the added advantage of being able to have an adequate number of students in order to form and consistently hold a group.

> Jason was fortunate. His school had a support group which—although unlabeled—had a significant number of young people who were trying to stay straight. Through AA and his participation in this support group, he was able to maintain his sobriety through the end of the school year, at which time he graduated from high school.

Community-Based Aftercare

Both outpatient and inpatient programs usually provide structured aftercare programs, which include educational and support sessions and may involve individual and family counseling. Self-help groups are another option for supporting adolescents once they have gone through inpatient or outpatient treatment. Nearly all treatment programs will help a young person find and make a transition to a self-help group within the community.

Self-Help Groups

Self-help groups, such as Alcoholics Anonymous, Narcotics Anonymous, Drugs Anonymous, Al-Anon, or Alateen, are a viable option for many young people. Attending a self-help group may be suggested as a first step, depending on the skills and resources of an adolescent. All of these programs are modeled after Alcoholics Anonymous, which began in 1935, and is based on 12 steps and 12 traditions. The 12 steps are a "group of principles, spiritual in their nature, which, if practiced as a way of life, can expel the obsession to drink and enable the sufferer to become happily and usefully whole. The 12 traditions outline the means by which AA maintains its unity and relates itself to the world about it, the way it lives and grows" (Alcoholics Anonymous World Services, Inc., 1980, p. 15).

Groups based on AA generally have the following in common:

- They provide closed meetings during which only its members attend. In these meetings, members share personal information and give each other support.
- They provide open meetings for anyone to attend. In these meetings, a leader or speaker shares experiences.
- They are anonymous and confidential. Members address each other by their first names and hold everything that is shared at the meeting in confidence.
- They are fellowships, with no rigid rules, no fees, and a minimum of organization.
- There are no written records kept of meetings or membership.
- They are not affiliated with any religion, even though many of the groups rely on the principle of a "higher power."
- They are not connected with any political position or with any treatment program.
- Members share their experiences, strength, and hope for each other.
- Many use sponsors, who are more experienced members who "adopt" a younger member and are available to help 24 hours a day.

The following provides a brief outline of several groups that address alcohol and other drug issues.

Alcoholics Anonymous (AA)

The primary purpose of AA is to establish and maintain sobriety for its members. The only requirement for membership in AA is the desire to stop drinking. AA is based on the belief that alcoholism is a progressive disease that has no cure. Abstaining and focusing on the 12-step program are seen as a way to begin recovery. Although AA has historically been focused on alcohol, increasing numbers of people have joined AA who are also addicted to other drugs. In smaller communities, AA may be the only self-help program available to help people cope with addiction. AA has traditionally been attended by adults; thus, some young people may feel out of place. Young people's AA meetings can be helpful; these are usually started and sponsored by adults in a community but attended almost exclusively by young people.

Narcotics Anonymous (NA)

NA is a self-help group for people who have a desire to stop using narcotics or other drugs, such as heroin, LSD, cocaine, crack, marijuana, barbiturates, amphetamines, and alcohol. Typically, more young people attend NA meetings, as the members are more often users of many drugs other than (or in addition to) alcohol and feel more comfortable talking about their addiction to other drugs at NA meetings.

Al-Anon

Al-Anon is a self-help group for families or friends of people who are dependent on alcohol or other drugs. Membership is open to young people as well as adults. Members follow the same general principles as do members of AA; they acknowledge that they are powerless over alcohol and that their lives have become unmanageable.

Alateen

Alateen is an affiliate of Al-Anon; Alateen recognizes that teenagers often do not feel comfortable talking about their feelings with adults. Alateen offers an atmosphere where adolescents can feel comfortable sharing their experiences with others their age.

Children of Alcoholics (COA)

Founded in 1983, COA groups are relatively new. COA groups provide support for children of people who are (or were) dependent on alcohol or other drugs. COA groups recognize that alcohol and other drug abuse is generational and affects children and other family members. Some COA groups are provided for young children and adolescents; Adult Children of Alcoholics (ACOA) groups often provide support for adults who grew up in homes where dependency created family problems.

How Could I Start a Student Assistance Program in My School?

If your school does not have a student assistance program, you can be instrumental in getting one started. Although you may not be the person who will be in charge of implementing the program, you can act as a catalyst by getting the information to the appropriate people and continuing to advocate for the program. The information in this part of the chapter is not intended to be a full guide for implementing a student assistance program. You will find resources in Appendix A. This information will simply provide an overview of the process of getting a program started and give you some steps to consider.

Get Support

If you are not the logical person to be in charge of a student assistance program, then your first step is to get support for the program from others in your school. To prepare, you might try running the idea of a student assistance program by one or two trusted colleagues or friends to find out their reactions. The next step is to identify others in the school who might be receptive and facilitate a meeting to discuss the idea. Eventually, you must gain administrative support. Only you can decide at which time in the process your school's administrators should be involved. Many administrators will be involved or take leadership of this program from the very start. Some will need to be convinced of its efficiency and effectiveness before they get behind the program.

Organize an Advisory Group

The task force or advisory committee for a student assistance program should minimally include representatives from the school administration (including your athletic administrator), teaching and cocurricular staff, support staff, special services staff (prevention specialist, social worker, psychologist, and school nurse), students, and parents. It may also include community representatives, such as law enforcement officials, assessment and treatment agencies, and other community representatives. This broad representation ensures that people who ultimately will be affected by the program will have a voice in its creation. It also makes later communication about the program easier.

Develop a Policy

The next step is to create a policy and get it approved by your school board. This policy should be brief and to the point. The policy gives direction for the program, a rationale for its existence, and permission for staff to act in accordance. It clearly specifies both the focus (problem-specific or broadbrush) and the scope (intervention or a combination of intervention, prevention, and health promotion). It does not get into specific procedures that might require continuous board review and approval to modify. Figure 10.2 gives an example of a broadbrush student assistance policy.

Establish Procedures

Student-assistance-program procedures spell out every step of the assistance process. Some of these procedures are eventually included in parent, student, and staff handbooks. In order to develop these procedures, other documents must be reviewed, such as discipline and attendance, athletic codes, and other educational policies and procedures. Together, these procedures generally cover the following areas:

- Identifying students
- The referral process (self-referral or referral from students, parents, and staff)
- How the student assistance program connects with other procedures and policies
- Interaction with other programs, such as special education

- Student assistance team functions
- Connection to a student's right to due process
- What to do in a crisis
- How school and community resources are to be used
- Confidentiality and data privacy
- Maintenance of student records
- Communication with parents
- Evaluating the program
- Helping students maintain academic progress during treatment
- Supporting students following treatment

Many students are troubled by problems which interfere not only with their academic and cocurricular performance but also with their emotional, physical, mental, and social development. The main goal of the student assistance program is to systematically and professionally respond to students' problems as they are manifested in school.

The student assistance program will provide a structured, organized approach to all schools within the district to offer assistance to students troubled by physical, emotional, social, legal, educational, sexual, medical, familial, or chemical-use problems. It will also provide a structured, organized liaison between the school and outside agencies. This includes monitoring the educational program of students in a treatment facility and assisting in the adjustment of a student returning from an outside placement.

1. This policy does not alter or replace existing administrative policy, disciplinary procedures, contractual agreements, or state law, but it does serve to assist in their utilization.
2. The policy applies to all students.
3. Students will be encouraged to seek assistance to determine if personal problems are causing unsatisfactory academic or cocurricular performance. If performance problems are corrected, no further action will be taken.
4. It is the intent of the student assistance program to work cooperatively with parents and guardians to resolve student problems. Parents and guardians will be contacted as soon as possible when appropriate.
5. All records and discussions of personal problems will be handled in a confidential manner. These records will be kept at the designated counseling resource and will not become a part of the student's cumulative file.
6. The program provides for preliminary assessment of student problems and referral, if appropriate. Costs for diagnostic and treatment services outside the school are the responsibility of parents or guardians.

This policy recognizes the responsibility of the school in responding to student problems. The school also recognizes its role and responsibility to prevent problems and promote health as a part of a comprehensive program.

Figure 10.2   Sample student-assistance policy.
Reprinted from Funk, Svendsen, Cunningham, and Griffin (1989).

Take Stock of In-School Resources

Resources may be available within the school to both prevent and respond to emotional, social, physical, and academic concerns. However, staff may not be aware of the resources that are available or the process by which students and their parents can access them. A coordinated student assistance program may also identify gaps in services or places where services overlap or duplicate each other. One of the first tasks of a student assistance program is to take a systematic and thorough inventory of the resources that are available within the school.

Develop Cooperative Relationships With Community Agencies and Organizations

Once the student assistance team has taken stock of the services available within the school, its next task is to identify resources in the community that can pick up where the school services end. Community resources need to be identified and catalogued to make sure that the needs of students and their families can be met when school resources are not appropriate or available. Student assistance teams can also help identify the types of funding needed for parents to access the services available, such as self-payment, insurance, company benefit plans, and local, county, state, or federal funds. Some schools are now working in collaboration with community agencies to locate services at or near a school, thereby cutting down on transportation and other barriers to help. Student assistance teams can help develop these cooperative relationships.

Create an Evaluation Plan

Each school's student assistance program has its own goals and objectives based on the concerns and needs of the school and community. These goals and objectives should be measurable so that the effectiveness of the student assistance program can be frequently monitored. This section briefly outlines some of the considerations for evaluating a student assistance program.

Outcome Evaluation

An evaluation plan should address the ultimate (long-range) outcome of a student assistance program: to prevent or reduce problems that interfere with learning. The long-range outcomes to be evaluated are dependent on the focus and scope of the student assistance program. Examples of possible outcomes that can be evaluated on a long-term basis (1-3 years) are

- improved attendance;
- reduced dropout rate;
- reduced classroom disruption;
- reduced incidents of verbal or physical violence;
- reduced tobacco, alcohol, or other drug use; and
- increased parental involvement.

Process Evaluation

On an annual basis, perceptions about the program and its implementation can be monitored through staff, parent, and student surveys on the following topics:

- Awareness of the student assistance program
- Knowledge of procedures
- Number of times staff members have talked with or referred a student
- Barriers to using the process
- Benefits of using the process
- Likelihood of staff members to document a student's behavior, to talk with a student about behavior, or to refer a student for assistance
- Staff members' perceptions of their own effectiveness in documenting behavior, talking with students about their behavior, or referring students for assistance
- Perception of the program's effectiveness

Short-Term Follow-Up

The evaluation plan should also specify how the program will be monitored on a more frequent basis. Items to be checked through a 60-day follow-up process include the following:

- Who referred the student? Referrals may come from a parent, another student, or a member of the school staff, such as a coach, teacher, counselor, school psychologist, school nurse, special education teacher, administrator, or speech teacher.
- How many self-referrals were made? This can be an indication of the students' perception of how helpful and confidential the program is.
- Why were the students referred? Some reasons include a violation of an athletic policy; low academic performance; behavioral concerns; mental-health concerns; speech and language difficulties; suspected child abuse; new-student adjustment; suspected or actual tobacco, alcohol, or other drug use or abuse; school policy violations; attendance problems; legal problems; or parental request.
- What happened with the referral? How many students did not require further services? How many did require further services, and for those, was the student referred to in-school or community-based resources?
- How many of the situations were able to be resolved to the satisfaction of the referent? In other words, how often did the behavior that resulted in the initial referral cease to be a concern to the referent?

Conduct Workshops for Staff, Students, and Parents

All staff, students, and parents need to know why the program was created, what its goals are, and how the program will help them.

They need to know how to make a referral to the program and what will happen once they have made a referral. Everyone also needs to know that information is kept strictly confidential and that no one will be penalized for being involved in the student assistance program (unless they have violated a school policy that has consequences and this violation triggers a referral). Staff, students, and parents need to have specific information in order to fully use the program.

Select and Train the Student Assistance Team

In addition, the student assistance team needs specialized training in assessment interviewing, intervention, referral, follow-up, use of community resources, and communication with families, students, and staff. They may also need further training in special areas that the student assistance program is designed to address.

Implement the Program

Once the previous steps have been taken, the program can be implemented. The student assistance team meets on a regular basis (weekly or biweekly) to respond to and monitor referrals, to identify and develop school and community resources, and to support students, parents, and staff as they make referrals to the program.

Evaluate and Revise the Program

With the team meeting on a regular basis, the program is self-correcting. Problems with the process are automatically identified, and the program is adjusted accordingly. The short-term (60-day) follow-up evaluation described earlier helps the team to monitor the number, types, and dispositions of the referrals received. An annual survey can determine perceptions about the program, and a long-term outcome evaluation can help to determine if the student assistance program is actually changing student behavior.

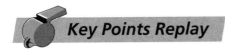 **Key Points Replay**

- The school, as an educational institution, is not an appropriate place to treat students who are dependent on alcohol and other drugs. However, the school can be instrumental in recognizing, referring, and supporting these students so they can participate fully in academic and cocurricular programs.

- Because of its limited resources, schools must develop strong relationships with community agencies that provide assessment, treatment, and aftercare for adolescents.

- Self-help groups, such as Alcoholics Anonymous, Narcotics Anonymous, and Drugs Anonymous are a viable option for many young people.

■ Athletes who live with someone who is experiencing problems with alcohol or other drugs have special needs. Al-Anon or Alateen, in-school support groups, and community family programs are options for these students.

■ If your school does not have a student assistance program, you can be instrumental in getting one started. Although you may not be the person who will be in charge of implementing the program, you can act as a catalyst in getting the information to the appropriate people and continuing to advocate the program.

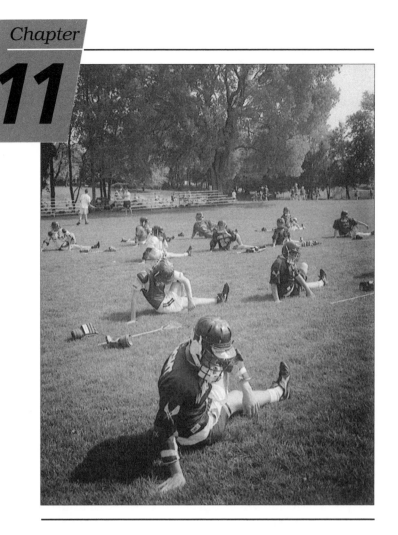

Chapter

11

Selecting Educational Resources

Chapter Warm-Up

Chapter 11 will help you identify other prevention resources that can be used. As discussed in Part I of *Coaches Guide to Drugs and Sport*, part of your role in prevention includes providing information about tobacco, alcohol, and other drugs by using teachable moments and preseason meetings. In addition, you may wish to conduct more formal educational sessions or use prepared educational materials to give information to your athletes or their parents. In chapter 11, you will learn how to plan these educational sessions, how to evaluate these educational materials, and how to involve others in helping you put these sessions together.

Planning for Educational Sessions

Before selecting materials or a program, it is important to clearly identify your purpose and objectives for the educational session. The planning considerations for conducting preseason meetings described in chapter 5 (pp. 62-65) are useful for planning any educational session and can be used as a starting point.

Purpose of Educational Sessions

Keeping your audience in mind can help to keep your prevention efforts focused. The overall goals of our educational efforts with athletes should be to

- reinforce the decisions of those who are currently not using tobacco, alcohol, or other drugs;
- encourage those who are experimenting with tobacco, alcohol, or other drugs to discontinue this behavior; and
- get those who are regular users of tobacco, alcohol, or other drugs to stop using and get help if they are having difficulty doing so.

When working with parents, we want them to support and work toward the above goals for athletes. Keep in mind that you will be working with parents who

- do not use tobacco, alcohol, or other drugs;
- use alcohol or prescription drugs appropriately, moderately, and legally; or
- misuse tobacco, alcohol, and other drugs or are dependent.

It will be difficult to target your messages toward this last group. If you include information like "Setting Personal Guidelines" discussed in chapter 3 (pp. 30-35), some of the parents in this group may be able to change their behavior. However, many in this group may see nothing wrong with their use, and may disregard your efforts. Do not be overly discouraged. Generally, this will be a very small percentage of your group. Your task will be getting others to support prevention efforts for young people and to work together on these efforts.

When talking about appropriate adult role modeling, you may find that the adult nonusers may think that people should never use tobacco, alcohol, and other drugs, and those adults who use appropriately, moderately, and legally may think that their way is the best way to deal with tobacco, alcohol, and other drugs. The goal is to keep this from being divisive; identify that both positions are attempting to avoid the problems that result from drug use, and work toward nonuse for young people who are under the legal limit.

A Case for Repetition

"Research About Drug Education" (chapter 5, pp. 56-59) noted that providing accurate information and repeating nonuse messages in combination with other strategies can be effective in preventing to-bacco, alcohol, and other drug use. Young athletes need repeated opportunities to learn and practice essential skills such as decision making and refusal skills. Parents need repeated opportunities to learn skills, too, such as setting limits and boundaries. Repetition or practice is also important for skill development. One-time prevention events generally have little long-term impact on behavior. Effective prevention is a series of activities and events.

In some prevention efforts, information is covered once, or skills are introduced; little or no time may be given for assimilating information or practicing skills. The skills may be taught generically, and it is expected that the students will be able to apply them to any one of several prevention areas, including areas such as drug use, violence, and sex. In fact, when a session is conducted that repeats information, reinforces a previously taught skill, or applies a previously taught skill to a different area, you may hear: "Oh, we did that last year," or "We did that in health class."

Lack of repetition or the opportunity to assimilate and practice can be compared to having athletes practice a skill only once or twice. We would not expect athletes to have much success in a sport with little or no practice. In sports, we repeatedly practice skills so that the skill becomes polished, improved, or permanent. For these same reasons, athletes need to hear prevention messages and practice the skills more than once. In addition, these prevention skills need to be practiced in the different situations in which they may be needed. We often put athletes into scrimmages and other simulated situations so that they can experience using a skill in the actual situation in which it might be used. The same is true for prevention skills. If we expect young people to use a refusal skill in a situation concerning tobacco, alcohol, and other drugs, they need to practice skills in that type of situation. If we expect them to use it in a situation involving violence, they should practice it in a simulated situation where violence is threatened.

As a coach, you understand the importance of repetition when instructing your athletes. You can provide and promote multiple opportunities for your athletes to hear accurate and consistent prevention information and to develop skills that will help them avoid using tobacco, alcohol, or other drugs.

Even though it is widely recognized and accepted that information alone is not likely to prevent [tobacco,] alcohol, and other drug problems, it is still a relatively important part of sending prevention messages.

Involving Others in Planning

Providing instruction in prevention skills may require the use of other resources in your school and community. Although you may be less directly involved in the instruction, you can provide—or encourage opportunities for—your athletes and their parents to be involved in programs which develop such skills and provide information. A student assistance coordinator and prevention specialists from drug programs in your school or community can help you plan and conduct your educational sessions, including selecting educational materials and programs. They can also help you determine how your efforts will fit with other prevention efforts taking place in the school and community. Your efforts should dovetail with other prevention efforts so that consistent messages about tobacco, alcohol, and other drugs are sent from many segments of the community.

Just as it is important to involve athletes and parents in the development of your athletic policies, you should include them when planning educational sessions. Athletes and parents can provide insight into current issues facing team members and their parents. Although there will probably be some topics you choose to address regardless of the interest expressed, the input of the athletes and parents can help you to tailor the content of your sessions so that the sessions are more relevant to the needs of athletes and their families. In addition, their involvement in the planning process can provide ownership, increasing active and positive involvement in these prevention efforts.

Some other people or organizations who could help you develop and conduct your educational sessions are

- other coaches of both high school and college sports,
- high school and college athletic administrators,
- school guidance counselors,
- school and community nurses,
- federal, state, and local law enforcement officials,
- sport psychologists,
- physicians,
- pharmacists,
- family therapists,
- county health educators,
- county and state alcohol and drug councils,
- private alcohol and other drug rehabilitation centers, and
- college or university staff specializing in addictions.

Your state department of education or state high school athletic or activity association may also be able to provide assistance. Appendix A lists some additional resources to help you develop or conduct educational sessions. Use the resources you have available in your school and community. Effective prevention requires that many segments of the school and community contribute to prevention efforts. Your athletes need to hear prevention messages from other segments of the community as well as their coach.

"To develop skills in appropriate behaviors is just like developing skills for athletic participation. You need to practice."

Malissa Martin

Potential Topics

Current trends about tobacco, alcohol, and other drug use among athletes and young people in general can give you direction for appropriate topics. If your school or community does periodic surveys on tobacco, alcohol, and other drugs, this is one source of information about current trends. Your state may conduct athlete or student surveys periodically. National surveys such as those regularly conducted by Johnston, O'Malley, and Bachman (1994) can provide general information about trends.

For instance, several sources indicate that there has been a progressive increase in the use of smokeless tobacco among young males. It also appears that the frequency of the use of many drugs by young females is increasing. These are examples of timely topics that could be tailored to specific audiences. Point out positive trends as well as negative ones.

The following are other topics that may be helpful to your athletes and other young people:

"Programs that allow athletes and parents to participate in its development are more likely to keep athletes and parents actively interested and participating."

Malissa Martin

- Identifying and counteracting social and personal influences that encourage the use of tobacco, alcohol, and other drugs
- Alternatives to using tobacco, alcohol, and other drugs
- Effects of tobacco, alcohol, or other drug use on athletic and academic performance
- Developing strength and endurance naturally
- Understanding choices and consequences
- Understanding dynamics of tobacco, alcohol, and other drug use in a family, team, or other group
- Getting help for problems with tobacco, alcohol, and other drugs
- How to use an assistance program
- Developing skills that will promote a positive and healthy lifestyle
- Developing positive leadership skills
- Developing self-worth outside of the athletic environment

Criteria for Selecting or Evaluating Educational Material

When selecting or evaluating educational resources, keep in mind the points listed under "Research About Drug Education" (chapter 5, pp. 56-59) as well as those listed below.

The following criteria are adapted from a report by the National Federation TARGET Program (1993a). The content of effective prevention material regarding tobacco, alcohol, and other drugs

- makes clear that all illegal drug use, including the underage use of alcohol and tobacco, is unhealthy and harmful for all persons;
- gives a clear message that risk is associated with using any form or amount of alcohol, tobacco, or other drugs;
- does not contain illustrations or dramatizations that could teach people ways to prepare, obtain, or ingest illegal drugs;
- does not glamorize or glorify the use of tobacco, alcohol, or other drugs;
- is cautious and careful about utilizing former drug users to provide prevention messages targeting youth; and
- recognizes the spectrum of tobacco, alcohol, and other drug use among young people and does not assume that all young people in a particular group use, use in a particular way, or have the same reasons for not using or using.

In addition, the content of effective prevention material regarding performance- or appearance-altering drugs, such as anabolic steroids,

- gives a clear message that any nonmedical use of steroids and other performance- and appearance-altering drugs is illegal and harmful to physical and emotional health;

- incorporates information designed to counter "win-at-all-costs" values and promotes the importance of participation, fun, and fair play in sports; and

- points out that the physiques of bodybuilders do not represent healthy or necessarily attractive ideals for young people to emulate.

Beyond the messages on tobacco, alcohol, and other drugs, check to see if the program or material fits the following guidelines.

Is Appropriate to the Target Audience

The material should match the target audience's cognitive and developmental levels, including reading and comprehension skills.

Uses Examples That Are Culturally, Ethnically, and Gender-Sensitive

While it is important to be sensitive to gender and different cultural backgrounds, it can be offensive to make general assumptions about a whole group of people. Even within groups, there is often a wide range of individual differences. Acknowledging individual and community differences as well as asking program participants to apply general principles to their own individual and community situations can keep you from making incorrect assumptions about individuals and groups.

Has a Credible Institutional Source

Make sure that the institution has experience in prevention education or research and that it does not have a significant vested interest in the outcome of its efforts. Several alcoholic beverage companies have developed prevention materials or have funded prevention programs. Some of these prevention programs have had their efforts questioned and have become embroiled in controversy because of this sponsorship.

Has a Credible Individual Source

If you hire a speaker or facilitator, make sure that person understands effective prevention concepts. Check out the person's experience in, and knowledge of, prevention education or research. Find out about the individual's interest in prevention or motives for being involved. Be careful of programs that are endorsed by those with celebrity status, especially athletes who are known users.

Uses Appropriate Language

The material or program should not use technical language or professional jargon that hinders understanding. The language and its messages should be consistent with generally accepted prevention principles. For instance, terms like "responsible use" should not be used, particularly when referring to young people. Also, avoid materials that use language that can be offensive to athletes and the various groups they represent.

Has a Respectful Tone

It is best if the tone of the material or program conveys that young people, including athletes, are valuable and capable persons, not problems that need constant supervision and guidance. The tone should not preach, moralize, or condescend to young people. The material or program can be strong on its emphasis of nonuse as the most appropriate choice for young people, but it should do so in a respectful manner.

Is an Appropriate Length

Your efforts to provide educational sessions for your athletes on tobacco, alcohol, and other drugs is to be commended. We recognize that prevention of tobacco, alcohol, and other drug use is not the primary purpose of athletic programs. Yet, as discussed in chapter 1, athletic programs provide a unique opportunity for prevention and educational sessions, and they can be an important part of prevention efforts. However, these efforts should not overwhelm athletes. Repeated, shorter sessions are more favorable than long, tedious sessions. When choosing programs and materials, including videos and films, it is preferable to choose those where passive listening or watching is short. Allow time for discussion. Also, be reasonable with yourself. Most coaches put in countless hours with their athletes. Although these sessions are important, they should not overwhelm you.

Uses Acceptable Formats and Graphics

The format should be understandable and easy to follow. The same is true of graphics. The quality of the graphics should be relatively high and should not distract your audience from the message or the presentation. In this age of computers and electronic media, young people and adults are accustomed to high-quality graphics.

Uses Messages That Are Appealing, Believable, and Effective

Too often materials or programs are selected by adults with their perspective of what would be good for young people and with little or no input from young people themselves. Find out how young people like the material or program. Ask a few of your athletes what they think and find out if the program has been pretested or evaluated.

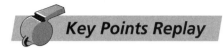

Key Points Replay

■ As a coach, you can use your influence to educate both your athletes and their parents about tobacco, alcohol, and other drugs by conducting preseason meetings and other educational sessions. Resources are available to help you conduct these sessions.

■ In order to plan effective educational sessions, it is important to clearly identify your purpose, objectives, and the outcomes you hope to achieve.

■ You will increase the effectiveness of these sessions if you involve others in planning your sessions, including school staff, athletes, and their parents.

■ As a coach, you use repetition and practice to help your athletes develop skills in sports. Repetition of information and opportunities to develop skills are equally important for prevention.

■ Your audience will likely have a broad spectrum of behaviors and feelings about tobacco, alcohol, and other drugs. Keeping this in mind will help you select topics and keep your prevention efforts focused.

■ Use established criteria for selecting and evaluating prevention programs, materials, and speakers. These criteria are based on what is effective in sending clear and consistent prevention messages; the criteria will help you increase the likelihood that the messages you send will be acceptable to, and appropriate for, your audience.

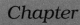

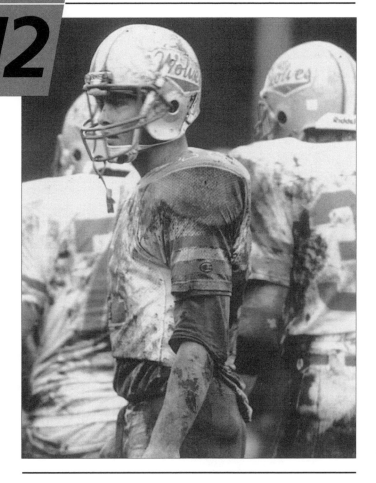

Drug Testing

Chapter Warm-Up

Chapter 12 will help you explore some of the possible benefits and drawbacks of drug testing, and it will examine some considerations concerning implementation of a drug-testing program.

In 1990, student athletes were tested for alcohol and 10 drugs in a school district south of Chicago. A lottery selected 15 athletes a week; during the semester a total of 277 athletes underwent screening. According to school officials, the testing cost between $40,000 and $50,000, which was paid through donations and increased ticket prices for football and basketball games.

On TARGET, April, 1990

Since the mid-1970s, when efforts to reduce drug use increased, drug testing of athletes has been used as a method of detecting controlled or illegal substances. Professional sports leagues, college athletic organizations, including the NCAA, and other amateur athletic programs, including the U.S. Olympic Committee, have considered and developed drug-testing programs as a method of responding to problems created by drug use among athletes.

Only 4% of those who responded to a Gallup poll conducted for the National Federation TARGET Program said their schools used drug testing as a part of their high school prevention program (National Federation TARGET Program, 1991). The National Federation of State High School Associations and its member state associations urge caution before embarking on a drug-testing program. Cost and litigation are two primary issues that should be given careful consideration.

Court cases have differed in their interpretation about the constitutionality of drug testing of student athletes at both the high school and collegiate levels. Court rulings have generally found random testing of students to be in violation of the Fourth Amendment's prohibition against unreasonable searches. In response, some schools have limited drug testing to student athletes because of the danger of injury to athletes who use drugs. Although two court decisions have ruled that random testing of student athletes violates their right to privacy ("Court Clouds Legality," 1994), in June 1995 the U.S. Supreme Court overturned a ruling that mandatory drug tests violate student athletes' privacy rights. These legal issues, as well as others discussed in this chapter, need to be seriously considered before instituting a drug-testing program.

Benefits of Drug Testing

Drug testing in athletics is usually intended to check for substances that could either provide an unfair advantage over those who do not use them or contribute to problems in the individual's life, including impaired athletic performance. People who have implemented drug testing believe that the following benefits will be realized by this approach.

Easier to Detect Drug Use Among Athletes

Usually athletes who use drugs are healthy and are not experiencing significant problems because of drug use. For some athletes, their superior physical abilities may mask any decline in performance. These factors may make detecting drug use difficult. With technological advances, drug testing can provide an additional and, sometimes, more definitive method of detecting the use of controlled or illegal substances.

May Be a Deterrent

The threat of positive detection and the resulting consequences may deter or prevent some individuals from using these substances. As covered in chapter 4, a rule has a more deterrent effect if there is consistent enforcement. Drug testing may boost the athletes' perceptions that they are likely to be found out if they violate a rule.

Levels the Playing Field

Testing for substances that may alter performance is done to ensure that competitive events are won or lost because of the physical and mental skills of the athletes rather than by an advantage gained from drug use. If drugs enhance performance, prohibiting their use and testing for them may be a way to eliminate the possible advantage that an opponent may gain by using them. Drug testing may also be a means of determining whether or not individuals are eligible to receive awards for a performance or to participate in future activities.

Identification and Referral

In other instances, drug testing may be used to identify and refer for appropriate help those individuals who may be having problems with the use of drugs. Some programs also use drug testing to ensure that an athlete remains free of the use of drugs after returning from a treatment program or after having been previously found to be using illegal drugs.

Drawbacks of Testing

Many of those who have implemented drug-testing programs—as well as those who have chosen not to—have identified the following drawbacks to drug testing.

Mixed Messages

Schools rarely test for all drugs, including tobacco and alcohol (the most commonly used drugs by adolescents). Focusing only on illicit drugs may give the message that these are the only drugs that concern the school. Testing for drugs based on a belief that drugs enhance performance can also send a mixed message. It may send the message that to perform better, an athlete should consider using performance-altering drugs.

Negative Reaction

Even those who are supportive of a prevention, education, or intervention program may be opposed to drug testing because they perceive that it violates an individual's rights. Some athletes say that drug testing makes them feel that they are guilty until they prove themselves innocent. Thus, testing may be viewed as a punitive measure for those suspected of use and is likely to be met with opposition.

Drug Testing Can Be Divisive

Consider how a drug-testing program can interfere with the underlying climate that you are working to establish through prevention efforts: a caring community, respect for students, and cooperation among staff, students, and families. Drug testing can create a barrier among athletes, their parents, and the school. Drug testing can pit administration and staff against students, as well as place the administration against coaches who do not believe in testing. Drug testing can set one group—athletes—against other groups in the school. Unless students who are involved in other cocurricular activities are tested, what are we saying about athletes? Are athletes more important than students who participate in other cocurricular activities? Do they have more problems than those who participate in other cocurricular activities? Unless we expand a testing program to include all students, are we saying that participants in cocurricular activities are more important than the entire student population?

Cost

Testing many students for all drugs is expensive. Funds may have to be diverted from other, more positive prevention approaches.

Labeling Athletes

People can come to the wrong conclusions based on the results of the tests—whether positive or negative. These erroneous conclusions can be harmful to individual athletes and your prevention efforts. When tests come back positive, people can make the assumption that an athlete is addicted to drugs. When tests come back negative, people can assume that the athlete is a nonuser. In fact, the only thing that these tests show is whether or not an athlete was using a particular drug during a particular time frame. For some drugs, such as alcohol, the time frame can be extremely short. If the majority of tests come back negative, the assumption can be made that there is no problem with drug use in athletics, and some people may be tempted to drop other prevention efforts.

Issues To Be Considered

In order to implement a drug-testing program, the following areas should be thoroughly explored by a committee of school board members, administrators, coaches, athletes, parents, student assistance team members, and community members. This may appear to be an onerous task, but it is essential. Often those who want to initiate drug testing do not consider all of its ramifications. As one athletic director said, "I don't really want to do drug testing, I just want my athletes to think I'm doing drug testing so it'll scare them away from doing any drugs."

Purpose

The effect you expect to achieve by instituting a drug-testing program should be clear. Determine if the focus of testing is to prevent the use of drugs, to intervene in drug use, or both. Hopefully, it is not just to scare kids away from doing drugs. Defining your purpose will help you decide for which drugs you will be testing and what policies, procedures, and programs need to coincide with the testing program. The purpose and outcome will affect the way you publicize and promote the program in the community.

Participants

Who will be tested through this program should be clearly identified and closely tied to the purposes for testing. Will all athletes be tested, or will the tests be done randomly? If random, how will the random sample be generated? Will just athletes be tested, or will others who participate in cocurricular activities? Or will all students be tested? If testing is done for ensuring fair competition or for safety in athletics, then testing is not necessary for all students; test only athletes and others involved in competitions that might be affected by drug use. These questions have legal implications and will also affect how favorably a testing program will be perceived in a community.

Frequency

Decide under what circumstances tests will be conducted. How many times per season or year will the tests be conducted? Will the tests be scheduled or unscheduled, announced or unannounced?

Costs

Estimate the cost of testing. If testing is to be comprehensive enough to detect many substances, including anabolic steroids, the cost of a single test may exceed $100, not including collection costs or retesting. You may be able to test for less, but the tests will not be as comprehensive, which may lead others to conclude that some drugs are acceptable, and others are not. With less expensive tests, the results might not be as accurate.

Procedures

One of the most difficult tasks is to develop exact procedures under which testing will be conducted. Faulty procedures can invalidate the findings of the tests. For instance, questionable collection of a specimen or a break in the chain of handling a specimen could lead to challenges of the test results. The individual tested can claim that the specimen was not hers or that it was contaminated.

Here are some questions to consider:

- How will testing procedures be communicated?
- How will participants be informed that they are to be tested?
- Who will collect specimens for testing?
- How will the specimens be collected?
- How will participants be observed during testing?
- How will specimens be handled?
- Who will analyze the specimens?

The National Collegiate Athletic Association (NCAA) has made a video that describes its drug-testing program and gives more information about drug-testing procedures (See Appendix A, p. 157 for NCAA address).

Results

It is essential to obtain informed consent from each individual to be tested, and each individual has a right to know how the results of the test will be used. Considering your purpose for the drug-testing program, you need to decide what you will do with the results. Here are some areas to explore:

- Who will be notified of the results? What will that person do with the information?
- How will the procedures differ if the results are negative or positive? Will you inform law-enforcement authorities if the test is positive?
- How will you verify the results?
- How will you protect the rights of the individual to confidentiality?

Connection to Other Programs and Policies

"Every community and school has its own wrinkles and twists. You must honor those twists and wrinkles to make prevention work."

Bill Mayo,
Athletic Director,
Blytheville, AK

Consider how a drug-testing program fits or conflicts with other school prevention and intervention efforts. How does the drug-testing program fit with the student assistance program? There should not only be consequences for confirmed positive tests, but there should be opportunities for help and assistance for troubled athletes. Also, consider how they will be educated about the effects, risks, benefits, and consequences of tobacco, alcohol, and other drug use. Drug-testing programs should never be implemented in the absence of comprehensive education and prevention efforts through athletics.

Drug testing has been implemented in some high schools because of very real fears about the implications of drug use and athletics. Communities have wanted to send a clear and strong message to high school athletes about drugs, and testing was seen as a way to emphatically do so. However, as different strategies and more positive approaches have evolved, been attempted, and found successful, reliance on drug testing as a prevention strategy has waned. In any event, drug testing, like codes of conduct, should only be a small part of other more extensive efforts.

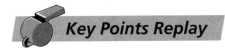

Key Points Replay

■ Only about 4% of the schools in the United States have implemented drug-testing programs at the high school level.

■ Even though the constitutionality of drug testing has been upheld by the U.S. Supreme Court, many coaches, parents, and students feel that drug testing is an invasion of privacy.

■ If drug testing is used, careful attention to policies and procedures can help reduce the negative reaction that can occur when drug-testing programs are implemented.

■ The effect of drug-testing programs on other prevention and intervention efforts should be considered.

■ If used, drug testing must be only one small part of a comprehensive prevention and intervention effort.

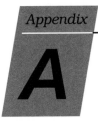

Appendix

A

Educational Resources

Educational Materials

This appendix lists print and audiovisual materials that may help you provide information that encourages athletes not to use alcohol, tobacco, and other drugs. The materials are grouped by those appropriate for both athletes and parents, primarily for student athletes, primarily for parents, and primarily for coaches and other school staff. In addition to a brief description, the source for ordering or obtaining further information is listed. The addresses and phone numbers of the sources can be found in on pp. 156-158.

Materials for Student Athletes and Parents

The materials listed below can be used with both athletes and their parents. You may also find these resources valuable to help you prepare for sessions with athletes or their parents.

Choosing Not To Use Alcohol: Benefits for Adolescents

"Because it's illegal!" is not enough to keep many adolescents from drinking alcohol. This trifold pamphlet goes beyond legality and offers adolescents, their parents, teachers, coaches, and other concerned adults concrete and easily understood examples of the benefits for adolescents to choose not to use alcohol. National Federation.

Operation Prom/Graduation

This guide presents a dynamic program filled with ideas to promote tobacco-, alcohol-, and other drug-free activities for students, particularly at high-risk times such as prom and graduation. National Federation.

Teaming for Prevention

This eight-page publication encourages parents, students, and their coaches and activity leaders to join forces to prevent tobacco, alcohol, and other drug problems. It gives practical suggestions about what these individuals can do, separately and together, to prevent problems. National Federation.

To Learn and To Lead

This 16-page guide is directed at high school activity participants and involves many aspects of the community in the mentoring process—elementary students, middle and junior high school students, high school students, college students, challenged individuals, professionals, and senior citizens. It provides specific ways high schools can use the mentoring process to positively interface with the community and offers suggested activities. National Federation.

Freedom of Choice—Steroids—You Make the Choice

This 52-page book not only addresses problems with steroid use but also gives a plan for increasing strength naturally through good nutrition, strength training, and other conditioning techniques. Iowa High School Athletic Association.

Questions About Series

Factual information about each of 12 drugs or drug categories (alcohol, cocaine, drugs, hallucinogens, marijuana, opiates, phencyclidine, sedatives-hypnotics, solvents-inhalants, steroids, stimulants, and tobacco) is provided on 8-1/2 × 11 inch masters for duplication. Minnesota Prevention Resource Center.

The Spitting Image Teleconference Video

A 90-minute video of the National Federation's teleconference to help state athletic or activity associations, school administrators, and coaches use their influence to prevent young people from using smokeless tobacco. Kevin Ringhofer and Martha Harding served as moderators of the teleconference. Although this video was primarily produced for adults, it also includes a segment specifically created for student athletes. National Federation.

Downfall: Sports and Drugs

This documentary profiles athletes whose athletic careers were destroyed by drugs. Scenes of the athletes performing are mixed with sobering interviews. Drug-free athletes who compete are also featured. It addresses alcohol and other drug use, including steroid use. A guide for this video is also available. This videotape may be available from your school's prevention coordinator or school media center. National Clearinghouse for Alcohol and Drug Information.

Let's Connect

This award-winning, 12-minute video consists of three scenes designed to stimulate discussion among students, parents, and adult leaders as they address issues of teenage alcohol use and parent-teen communication. There are facilitator guides provided for each of the three scenes. National Federation.

The Rally: A Uniting of Students, Parents, and School Personnel to Address Issues of Alcohol and Other Drugs

This 28-minute video portrays some problems created by alcohol, tobacco, and other drug use by students and also documents the resulting discussions that bring coaches, parents, and student groups together to establish parameters for addressing tobacco-, alcohol-, and other drug-use issues. National Federation.

Materials for Student Athletes

The materials listed below are primarily targeted toward students and have appropriate topics and messages for student athletes. You may also find some of these resources helpful when preparing for sessions with your athletes.

If You Use Steroids, These Aren't the Only Things Stacked Against You

This brochure lists the negative effects of anabolic-androgenic steroids on the body. National Clearinghouse for Alcohol and Drug Information.

Everyone a Hero

The premise of this program, developed by the Colorado High School Activities Association (in conjunction with the authors of this book), is to use the strongest asset in high schools—their students—to serve as role models and to deliver a consistent message to younger students in elementary, middle, and junior high schools. High school students talk about high school life, their commitment to extracurricular activities, and their decisions not to use tobacco, alcohol, and other drugs. A video and 35-page companion teaching guide instruct the high school students on how they can present this nonuse message to younger students. National Federation.

Narc

This 26-minute video presents the dilemma that arises when a popular and accomplished high school student tries to prevent an athlete from driving while drunk. This engaging drama presents important lessons about alcohol misuse, the temptations of following the crowd, and the difficulties and benefits of standing up for your beliefs. Films for the Humanities and Sciences.

The Spitting Image: Is Chewing Tobacco a Part of the Game?

This four-page brochure covers the effects and risks of smokeless tobacco use while pointing out the benefits to athletes of being "spit-free." National Federation.

Steroids—To Use or Not To Use? A Guide for Students

This pamphlet offers students valuable and honest information about the effects and risks of steroid use. Suggestions for resisting influences to use steroids and alternative ways to improve performance are provided in clear and straightforward language. Companion pieces for parents (p. 153) and coaches (p. 155) are also available. National Federation.

Sports United Against Drugs

This resource guide and video are directed at athletes to support drug education and prevention programs. A 16-page booklet includes tips on preparing and delivering presentations and instructions to help athletes deliver factual information on alcohol, other drugs, and other lifestyle issues. A 13-minute video features high school students in a documentary discussion, along with clips of prominent athletes delivering messages about what can be accomplished by setting the proper goals, motivation, and hard work. National Federation.

Students and Steroids—The Facts Straight Up

This kit contains a classroom curriculum featuring two 14-minute videos, complete instructor's guide, and activities. It also has a special summary video for parents and coaches as well as motivational posters. Topics include how a person can get stronger without using steroids, the advantages of a drug-free lifestyle, and the warning signs of steroid use. National Federation.

Tips for Teens Series

This series of brochures (on alcohol, smoking, crack and cocaine, marijuana, and hallucinogens) provides facts and dispels myths about tobacco, alcohol, and other drug use. Each brochure provides information on long- and short-term effects, physical and psychological risks, and legal implications. These brochures are printed on brightly colored paper and designed in an interesting and abstract manner to attract the attention of teens. A list of resources is provided. National Clearinghouse for Alcohol and Drug Information.

No Matter How You Say It, Say No

Developed by the Department of Health and Human Services in conjunction with the National Basketball Association, this 11-minute video features former Detroit Piston Isiah Thomas visiting with young people and discussing the pressures to use alcohol and other drugs. Thomas gives them reasons for not using drugs and explains steps to refuse drugs without alienating friends. Most appropriate for junior high school students. Companion pieces for students (p. 152) are also available. National Federation.

Materials for Parents

The materials listed below are most appropriate for parents and other adults.

Steroids and Our Students: A Guide for Parents

This pamphlet is a short, easy-to-read guide for helping parents learn how they can influence their children to avoid the use of steroids. The information addresses health, safety, and ethical reasons for not using steroids and emphasizes the important role of parents in preventing steroid use. Companion pieces for students (p. 152) and coaches (p. 155) are also available. National Federation.

Responsible Hosting: Some Suggestions for Entertaining with Alcohol

This four-page brochure provides hosting tips for the moderate and appropriate use of alcohol, responsible attitudes about alcohol, and some recipes for nonalcoholic drinks. Minnesota Prevention Resource Center.

Non-Alcoholic Party Drinks

This 35-page booklet provides guidelines for appropriate and moderate use of alcohol, hosting tips, and many recipes for nonalcoholic beverages and appetizers. Minnesota Prevention Resource Center.

Materials for Coaches and Other School Staff

The materials listed below can help you prepare for sessions with athletes or their parents.

What, When, and How To Talk to Students About Alcohol and Other Drugs—A Guide for Teachers

This 86-page book discusses the role of the school and staff in developing prevention and student assistance programs. It discusses what kind of information students need at different ages and stages of development. It also gives discussion questions and role-playing vignettes, student outcomes by which to design or judge curricula, and school policy suggestions. Hazelden.

Preseason Meeting Handbook

This 24-page handbook guides coaches, athletic directors, activity sponsors, principals, school coordinators, and others through the preseason meeting process. It contains facts and findings to support activity programs and funding efforts, sample invitations, sample newspaper articles, and public service announcements. It also includes examples of agendas for a general information meeting and an individual sport meeting, as well as a sample student participant contract to not use tobacco, alcohol, and other drugs. National Federation.

Preseason Meeting Video

A 60-minute video of the National Federation TARGET's Preseason Meeting Satellite Broadcast shows schools how to orchestrate the preseason meeting. National Federation.

Student Assistance Program: How It Works

This 54-page book describes the broadbrush approach to student assistance. It explains the appropriate role of the school in responding to student problems and gives samples of actual policies, programs, and materials. Hazelden.

Student Assistance Model: The Response Component

This 50-page manual provides step-by-step guidance for implementing a student assistance program. It delineates the roles and responsibilities of a student assistance team and school staff members. It contains a particularly helpful appendix that gives flowcharts, sample policies, and actual forms that can be used to implement a program. Hazelden.

Playing Fair, Keeping Fit, Looking Good Without Using Steroids: A Guide to Preventing the Use of Steroids and Other Performance- and Appearance-Altering Drugs

This resource guide report provides information about problems with, and prevention strategies for, steroids and other performance- or appearance-altering drugs. The material is the result of the national summit conference sponsored by the National Federation TARGET Program. National Federation.

Preventing Adolescent Use of Anabolic Steroids

This package, composed of a 35-minute video and notebook materials, including facilitator or self-study guide, lecture or information notes, and activities, is designed to train coaches, athletic directors, and athletic trainers on their role in preventing anabolic-androgenic steroid and other drug use. Materials are available as a workshop kit or as a self-study course. National Federation.

Steroids and Our Students: A Guide for Coaches

This concise pamphlet offers coaches helpful information on the health, legal, and ethical risks of steroid use. Companion pieces for students (p. 152) and parents (p. 153) are also available. National Federation.

Steroids and Our Students: A Program Development Kit

The 70-page *Program Development Guide*, provided in a three-ring notebook, is designed to help athletic directors, coaches, and school administrators develop and implement policy and programs to prevent the use of steroids. National Federation.

Steroids: A Resource Guide

This 33-page guide contains information about the history, reasons, social influences, and risks of steroid use. It is a resource that can supplement prevention programs and can aid in the development of steroid prevention curriculum and activities. New York State Education Department.

Steroids

This brochure, designed for use by coaches, addresses the dangers of steroid use by America's young people. It is available in sets of 100, while quantities last, at no charge when ordered with other National Federation TARGET items. National Federation.

Educational Resource Organizations

Listed below are organizations that develop or provide educational resources on tobacco, alcohol, and other drugs. In addition, many state athletic or activity associations have resources and programs on tobacco, alcohol, and other drugs. Many state departments of education also have excellent resources and programs. If you need help contacting your state association or state department of education, contact the National Federation TARGET Program or the National Clearinghouse for Alcohol and Drug Information for assistance.

National Federation of State High School Associations TARGET Program

11724 N.W. Plaza Circle
P.O. Box 20626
Kansas City, MO 64195-0626
800-366-6667
816-464-5400

The National Federation TARGET Program provides information on preventing tobacco-, alcohol-, and other drug-use problems and on other healthy lifestyle issues surrounding high school athletics and activities. TARGET is the Center for Substance Abuse Prevention's designated Regional Alcohol and Drug Awareness Resource (RADAR) Specialty Center for the prevention of steroid and other performance- or appearance-altering drug use. The National Federation catalog contains descriptions and price information on print and audiovisual resources pertaining to healthy-lifestyle issues.

National Clearinghouse for Alcohol and Drug Information (NCADI)

P.O. Box 2345
Rockville, MD 20847-2345
800-729-6686

The NCADI has a free catalog containing information on a wide variety of low-cost materials regarding tobacco, alcohol, and other drugs. NCADI also provides access to the Prevention Materials Database, an on-line computer collection of prevention products. Its Prevention Pipeline, a bimonthly information service, gives information about research, resources, and activities in the prevention field. Grant applications and information about grant programs can also be obtained through NCADI.

Other Resource Organizations With Information About Sports and Drugs

American College of Sports Medicine

Box 1440
Indianapolis, IN 46206-1440
317-637-9200, Public Information

Drug Enforcement Administration

Demand Reduction Section
U.S. Department of Justice
Washington, DC 20537
202-307-7939, Public Affairs
202-307-7960, Demand Reduction Office

Films for the Humanities & Sciences

P.O. Box 2053
Princeton, NJ 08543-2053
800-257-5126

Harding, Ringhofer & Associates, Inc.

2200 Indian Road West
Minnetonka, MN 55305
612-545-4011

Hazelden Educational Materials

P.O. Box 176
15251 Pleasant Valley Rd.
Center City, MN 55012-0176
800-328-9000, outside of Minnesota
800-257-0070, Minnesota residents
612-257-4010, general number

Iowa High School Athletic Association (IHSAA)

P.O. Box 10
1605 S. Story
Boone, IA 50036-0010
515-432-2011

Minnesota Prevention Resource Center (MPRC)

2829 Verndale Ave.
Anoka, MN 55303
612-427-5310
800-247-1303, in Minnesota

Minnesota State High School League

2100 Freeway Blvd.
Brooklyn Center, MN 55430
612-560-2262

National Collegiate Athletic Association (NCAA)

6201 College Blvd.
Overland Park, KS 66211-2422
913-339-1906

National Strength and Conditioning Association

530 Communications Circle
Ste. 204
Colorado Springs, CO 80905
719-632-6722

New York State Education Department

Attn. Gail Harding
Mid-South Field Service Team
Albany, NY 12234
518-486-6054

Parents Resource Institute for Drug Education (PRIDE)

10 Park Pl. South
Ste. 340
Atlanta, GA 30303
404-577-4500
800-487-7743

Funding Resources

Many of the organizations listed above can direct you to available funds for preventing tobacco, alcohol, and other drug use through athletics. In addition, you may wish to contact the Center for Substance Abuse Prevention (CSAP) for procedures to request technical assistance, training, or information about funds:

Center for Substance Abuse Prevention
Rockwall II
9th Floor
5600 Fishers Ln.
Rockville, MD 20857
800-729-6686

Most of the strategies suggested in *Coaches Guide to Drugs and Sport* do not require extensive funds. For small projects, we suggest that you work with your local service organizations or your booster club to obtain funding. Your student athletes, particularly those who have shown positive leadership in the community, can readily obtain dollars for worthy projects by addressing a monthly meeting of a local service group.

Reference Guide to Common Drugs

Detailed knowledge about specific drugs is not essential for a coach to help prevent or respond to tobacco, alcohol, and other drug use. However, the information below may help to answer some questions you or your athletes have about various drugs. For information about the frequency of use of many of these drugs, refer to "The Extent of Tobacco, Alcohol, and Other Drug Use Among Athletes," pp. 7-13.

The following categories do not list dependency, tolerance, and withdrawal as either short- or long-term consequences of these drugs. Most of these drugs taken in sufficient quantity over a long enough time will produce dependency—physical, psychological, or both. The quantity and length of use needed to produce addiction varies with both the drug and the individual. Psychological dependency is probably the most serious. Most people can withdraw from a physically addictive drug within 24 hours to 2 weeks, depending on the individual and the drug; recovery from psychological dependency takes much longer. If this were not true, all we would have to do to treat dependency would be to provide physical detoxification. Instead, treatment for dependency requires attention to the physical, emotional, social, psychological, and spiritual aspects of the disease.

Note. Much of the following information is adapted from the "Questions About" series of fact sheets produced and distributed by the Minnesota Prevention Resource Center, 1995; funded by the Minnesota Department of Human Services; copyright 1990, 1995 by Minnesota Department of Human Services. Used with permission.

Drug name	What is it?	How is it used?
Alcohol	Alcohol (or ethanol) is contained in beer, wine, or distilled liquor. It is produced from the fermentation of fruits, vegetables, and grains; it contains calories and can be classified as food.	Alcohol is consumed as a beverage. It may be drunk as packaged (usual for beer and wine) or mixed with other beverages, such as soda or water. Alcohol is absorbed into the bloodstream in the stomach and small intestine. Alcohol is one of the most commonly used drugs among most groups of people in the United States.
Amphetamines (stimulant)	Amphetamines in pure form are yellowish crystals. On the street, they generally come in pill form and go by such names as "speed," "white crosses," "uppers," "dexies," "bennies," and "crystal."	Tablets or capsules are swallowed. The pure crystal form can also be sniffed or injected.

Short-term effects	Long-term effects and other health risks	Connection to athletics
Factors that influence the effects include the amount of alcohol, the rate at which it is consumed, the presence, amount, and kind of food in the stomach, weight, mood, and previous experience. In small amounts, alcohol has a tranquilizing effect on most people. However, it appears to stimulate some people, which may be the result of depressing certain parts of the brain and, thus, relaxing inhibitions. Moderate amounts of alcohol also affect other areas of the brain, resulting in flushing, dizziness, dulling of the senses, impaired coordination, reflexes, memory, and judgment. Larger quantities of alcohol may result in staggering, slurred speech, double or blurred vision, dulled senses, sudden mood changes, and unconsciousness.	Large quantities taken over a long period of time can damage the liver, heart, and pancreas. Malnutrition, gastrointestinal irritation, lowered resistance to disease, and irreversible nervous-system damage (including brain damage) can result. Several of these factors can lead to early death. Large amounts of alcohol ingested on a single occasion can lead to death due to depression of the brain areas that control breathing and heart rate.	Alcohol may be used by some athletes to help them relax prior to a contest or event. However, it is much more frequently used by athletes to relax or socialize after a contest or event.
Amphetamines stimulate the central nervous system, increasing alertness, speech, and activity. Increased energy is sensed by the user. Heart and breathing rates and blood pressure increase. Appetite decreases. Higher doses may increase the effects so that the user feels excitement and a greater sense of self-confidence and power. The user may also be restless and talkative. A dry mouth, fever, sweating, headache, blurred vision, dizziness, and sleeplessness may also occur. With very high doses, anxiety, irritability, paranoia, and even panic and hallucinations can occur.	Long-term use can result in weight loss, lack of sleep, malnutrition, skin disorders, vitamin deficiencies, and ulcers. Chronic users may develop an amphetamine psychosis, which includes seeing, hearing, and feeling things that do not exist, irrational thoughts or beliefs, and a feeling that people are out to get them. Sudden increases in blood pressure from an amphetamine injection may lead to death. Injecting amphetamines with unsterile equipment can increase the user's risk of infections, including HIV/AIDS and hepatitis. Self-prepared solutions can become contaminated, and injecting them may lead to lung disease, heart disease, and other diseases of the blood vessels, which may lead to death. Kidney and other tissue damage can also occur.	Because of the stimulant effects, amphetamines may be used by athletes to increase alertness, aggressiveness, endurance, and weight loss.

Drug name	What is it?	How is it used?
Amphetamines (stimulant) *(continued)*		
Barbiturates (sedative hypnotic)	Barbiturates are white powders sold as capsules, tablets, suppositories, or in liquid form.	Barbiturates are taken in the usual manner for the substance in which it is found: capsules, tablets, and suppositories. In liquid form they can be swallowed or injected. They are used to treat anxiety, tension, sleeplessness, and illnesses in which seizures and convulsions occur.
Benzodiazepines (sedative hypnotic)	Benzodiazepines include such drugs as Valium, Librium, and Xanax. They are sometimes referred to as minor tranquilizers. They are manufactured as capsules and tablets of many sizes, shapes, and colors.	Benzodiazepines capsules and tablets are usually taken orally. They have a calming effect without slowing the body down too much. They are used to reduce the anxiety and tension caused by stressful situations and emotional problems.

Short-term effects	Long-term effects and other health risks	Connection to athletics
	Look-alike amphetamines can also present some serious health risks. They usually contain some amount of a legal stimulant often found in over-the-counter diet pills and decongestants, but they are sold on the street and are marked like speed or uppers. Because these look-alike drugs are less potent than speed or uppers, there is a great deal of risk for users of look-alike drugs who, intentionally or accidentally, take the same amount of real amphetamines.	
Small doses of barbiturates relax muscles and reduce anxiety and tension, leading to calmness. Larger doses act like alcohol to produce slurred speech, staggering, poor judgment, and slow, uncertain reflexes.

Much larger doses may cause unconsciousness and death. Only a small difference exists between a dose that results in sleep and one that results in death; therefore, those who are given prescription barbiturates need to be directed to take only the amount prescribed. | These drugs are particularly dangerous if taken in combination with other drugs that slow down the body, like alcohol. Effects are multiplied, and the risk of slowing down breathing to the point of death greatly increases. The use of barbiturates and alcohol together is the most common method of overdose that results in death. Regular use over time can produce a tolerance. As the user takes larger and larger doses to get the same effect, the difference between a dose that produces sleep and one that results in death decreases. | Athletes are likely to use barbiturates for the same reasons other users would. There may be a tendency to use barbiturates to reduce the anxiety related to competition and to help athletes sleep better because of the stress of competition. |
| Low doses of benzodiazepines can relieve mild anxiety, tension, and nervousness with little effect on the user's mental or physical functioning. A sense of relaxation and well-being will occur for some users. Others may feel drowsy or out of touch, so their doctor will adjust the dosage.

Higher doses may cause drowsiness and impair coordination. These drugs affect the way the mind perceives things and how the mind and muscles work together. A user should not drive or operate machinery. | Tolerance may develop slowly over a long period of time. Withdrawal symptoms include sweating, stomach cramps, nervousness, tremors, and convulsions. | Although athletes are likely to use benzodiazepines for the same reasons other users would, there may be a tendency to use benzodiazepines to reduce the anxiety related to competition and to help athletes sleep better because of the stress of competition. |

Drug name	What is it?	How is it used?
Caffeine (stimulant)	Caffeine is a white, bitter, crystal-like substance found in coffee, tea, cocoa, and cola. It is also found in some products such as aspirin, nonprescription cough and cold medicines, soft drinks, diet pills, and some street drugs. Caffeine may be the world's most popular drug.	It is usually consumed orally in the substance in which it is found: beverages, pills, or liquid medicines and drugs. In rare cases, it may be used in a suppository form. It is often used to provide energy for the user.
Cocaine (stimulant)	Cocaine is a white powder produced from the leaves of the South American coca plant. A smokable form of cocaine is called "crack" because of the crackling sound it makes when smoked.	It can be inhaled, sniffed, injected, or smoked.

Short-term effects	Long-term effects and other health risks	Connection to athletics
Caffeine stimulates the central nervous system, increasing alertness and activity. The effects of 150 to 300 mg of caffeine (approximately two cups of coffee) begin in 15 to 30 minutes. There may be an increase in the user's general metabolism, body temperature, and blood pressure. Urine production and blood sugar levels may also increase.	Impaired coordination, hand tremors, decreased appetite, trouble sleeping, and boredom may result from chronic use of caffeine. Calcium absorption can be reduced with caffeine consumption. This could create bone density problems, especially for adolescents and females. Some studies link increased fibrocystic breast tissue in females to caffeine consumption. This could make it more difficult to detect lumps in breast examinations.	Caffeine may produce a stimulant effect, a general feeling of alertness, or a high which might help athletic performance. It may also increase endurance by altering the way sugars and fats are used during longer-lasting physical activities. However, the amount needed and the effect that this amount taken orally has on the digestive system can usually negate or override these possible positive effects. To negate these effects on the digestive system, some athletes use caffeine suppositories.
Very high amounts of caffeine may cause nausea, diarrhea, sleeplessness, trembling, headaches, and nervousness.	Individuals who suddenly stop using caffeine may experience withdrawal effects, including headaches, irritability, and mood changes.	
	Consuming poisonous doses of caffeine is rare, but they may result in convulsions and breathing failure. It is almost impossible to consume a poisonous dose by drinking coffee, tea, or soft drinks. However, deaths have been reported due to the use of tablets containing caffeine.	
Cocaine stimulates the central nervous system, resulting in increased alertness and activity. It increases blood pressure, heart rate, breathing rate, and body temperature. Blood vessels constrict, and pupils dilate. Use may cause a runny nose, loss of appetite, and sleep problems.	With continued use, the initial euphoric high is often gradually replaced with anxiety, irritability, and restlessness. The regular cocaine user may become confused or depressed. Violent or paranoid behavior, known as "cocaine psychosis," can result from cocaine use. While first-time users may experience cocaine psychosis, this mental condition occurs more rapidly in crack users and more frequently in regular cocaine users. Cocaine is very addictive. Crack users appear to be less willing or able than other cocaine users to control their use, indicating that crack use may result in strong psychological dependence.	The initial effect on athletic performance may be an increased sense of awareness and a high which could result in improved performance, or these feelings could just give the user a perception of better performance. Because the high is relatively short and followed by a low, performance may be negatively affected.
As the high usually experienced with use wears off, a severe low follows. These highs and lows are often more accentuated in crack use. The lows often leave the user craving more of the drug.		

Drug name	What is it?	How is it used?
Cocaine (stimulant) *(continued)*		
Hallucinogens and Psychedelics	Hallucinogens or psychedelics are a group of drugs that dramatically affect the user's perceptions. LSD, mescaline, MDMA (3.4-methylenedioxymethamphetamine) or ecstasy, psilocybin, and DMT (dimethyltryptamine) are some of the drugs in this group. LSD is partly made for lysergic acid. It is also found in ergot and the fungus which grows on rye and other grains. Mescaline comes from the peyote cactus. Psilocybin comes from certain mushrooms. What is sold on the street as mescaline or psilocybin is often LSD or PCP (phencyclidine). MDMA is structurally similar to methamphetamine and mescaline. DMT acts like LSD, but is shorter acting; it is sometimes referred to as the "businessman's trip." DMT effects begin almost immediately and last for 30 to 60 minutes. Designer drugs are also being manufactured in clandestine laboratories and marketed under the names of MDA, MMDA, and MDEA. These are analogues of amphetamines and methamphetamines and have similar effects.	These drugs are generally tablets or capsules and, occasionally, liquids. They are usually taken orally, but they can be sniffed, smoked, or injected. (There is no evidence that LSD comes in a tattoo form—a piece of paper laced with LSD—which is stuck to the skin and absorbed by the body. The paper would have to be treated with a very expensive amount of LSD to produce a high.)

Short-term effects	Long-term effects and other health risks	Connection to athletics
	The impact of cocaine on the nervous and cardiovascular systems may result in seizure, stroke, heart arrhythmias, or respiratory failure, any of which could be fatal. Users who inject cocaine with unsterile needles are at risk of getting tetanus, hepatitis, tuberculosis, or HIV/AIDS.	
The effects of these drugs vary greatly from user to user, depending upon on the dose amount; the user's personality, mood, and expectations; and the situation in which the drug is used. Effects usually are felt within 30 to 90 minutes after ingesting. Typical responses are dilated pupils; increased body temperature, heart rate, and blood pressure; sweating; loss of appetite; sleeplessness; dry mouth; and tremors. MDMA also stimulates the central nervous system, and users may also experience muscle tension, nausea, blurred vision, fainting, and chills. The user often experiences feelings of euphoria, well-being, and the sense of having great wisdom and insight. They may experience several different emotions at once or swing rapidly from one emotion to another. The user's sense of time and self are altered. Users may perceive a mix or crossover of sensations, such as hearing colors or seeing sounds. Boundaries may seem less distinct, so the user seems to blend in with the surroundings. To some, this may be pleasant, while for others it can be frightening. Unpleasant reactions ("bad trips") are common with these drugs and may last from a few minutes to several hours.	Flashbacks (parts of the original drug experience that recur without simultaneous use the drug) may be one effect of these drugs. However, they are rare and are more likely to occur with frequent use. After the use of psychedelic drugs, some users have experienced abnormal thought processes and disorganized personalities. However, these users often have a history of—or were likely to have—mental and emotional problems, so the exact relationship between the drug use and the emotional problem is not known.	The effects of hallucinogens would not seem to lend themselves to any particular athletic use. Athletes are most likely to use these drugs for the same reasons other users would.

Drug name	What is it?	How is it used?
Hallucinogens and Psychedelics *(continued)*		
Inhalants and Solvents	Most chemicals in this group are solvents derived from fossil fuels such as gasoline, paint and paint thinner, glue, nail polish remover, cleaning and lighter fluid, typewriter correction fluid, refrigerant gases, and aerosol products. The most frequently misused solvents are toluene, acetone, methyl and ethyl ketoses, benzene, xylem, hexane, freons, nitrous oxide, and volatile nitrates.	Inhalants are inhaled by sniffing through the nose or "huffing" through the mouth. Butyl and isobutyl nitrites are sold over the counter under a variety of names, such as Banaplle Gas, Locker, Rush, and Bolt. Nitrous oxide is used as a propellant in whipped cream, as a leak detector, or in dispensing machine "whippets." These whippets are metal cylinders containing nitrous oxide that can be purchased over the counter.

Short-term effects	Long-term effects and other health risks	Connection to athletics
These reactions may unmask hidden mental or emotional problems. Previously existing fears often become greater. The user may experience panic, confusion, paranoia, anxiety, unpleasant sensory images, feelings of helplessness, and loss of control.		
Immediate effects can be loss of the sense of pain or mental or physical excitement. A loss of consciousness and death can occur. A high lasts only 15 minutes to 1 hour. Solvents are very fat soluble. Absorption of solvents into fatty tissues can disrupt the normal functioning of organs like the brain, lungs, heart, liver, and certain blood cells. Too much solvent in the blood can slow down breathing and circulation. Nausea, vomiting, and fainting can result, especially with butyl and isobutyl nitrite use.	Death may result from suffocation, heart attack, or accidents. Because solvents are very fat soluble and not water soluble, it may take two weeks or longer for these substances to be completely eliminated from the body. Chronic use of inhalants or solvents can inhibit one's ability to think clearly, to remember things, to determine right from wrong, and to solve problems. It can destroy brain and nerve cells, and it can damage the lungs, heart, liver, kidneys, throat, nasal passageways, teeth, and gums. Users often withdraw from activities, and they may become depressed or violent. Severe mood swings may occur, along with a loss of appetite, tiredness, nausea, headaches, chapped or reddened skin about the nose and mouth, and nosebleeds. Excessive use of the nitrites may cause damage to the heart, blood vessels, and immune system. Those who misuse nitrous oxide over a long period of time may experience loss of balance, leg weakness, tingling and numbness in the fingers and toes, and other nerve damage. Shortness of breath, nausea, irregular heartbeat, and hearing loss are also experienced by some users.	The effects of inhalants or solvents would not seem to lend themselves to any particular athletic use. Athletes are most likely to use these drugs for the same reasons other users would.

Drug name	What is it?	How is it used?
Marijuana	Marijuana is the common name for the hemp plant, cannabis sativa. THC (Delta-9-tetrahydro-cannabinol) is the primary mind-altering chemical in marijuana, and most of it comes from the flowering tops of the plant. Plant strain, climate, soil conditions, time of harvesting, and other factors determine the potency of marijuana. Potency of marijuana today is generally much stronger, up to 10 times, than it was 20 years ago. Grass, pot, weed, and chronic are some other names used for marijuana. Hashish or "hash" is made by extracting the resin from the leaves and flowers of the plant and pressing it into cakes or slabs. Hash usually contains 5 to 10 times as much THC than crude marijuana. Hash oil may contain up to 50% more THC.	Marijuana in its various forms is usually smoked in a rolled cigarette paper ("joints" or "reefers"), pipes, or a "blunt," which is a small cigar that is emptied and refilled. Sometimes it is baked into foods and eaten. It takes longer for the user to experience the short-term effects of marijuana when it is eaten.
Opiates	Opiates are a group of drugs that reduce pain and promote sleep. Opium, morphine, heroin, and codeine are opiates that come from the juice of the Asian poppy's seed pod. Opioids are synthetic drugs chemically related to opiates. Opium is a dark brown substance that may be available in chunks or a powder. Heroin is a whitish or brownish powder. Street heroin is usually cut (diluted) with sugar, quinine, or other substances. Other opiates come in a variety of forms, such as capsules, tablets, syrups, solutions, and suppositories.	Opium is usually smoked or eaten. Heroin is usually dissolved in water to be injected as a liquid. Other opiates are taken in the usual manner for the substance in which it is found: capsules, tablets, syrups, solutions, and suppositories.

Short-term effects	Long-term effects and other health risks	Connection to athletics
Immediate effects of marijuana use are increased heart rate, bloodshot eyes, dryness in the mouth and throat, and relaxation. A decreased ability to do tasks which require concentration, reaction time, and coordination can result from impaired memory and an altered sense of time from marijuana use. Some users may experience panic attacks, usually described as an exaggeration of the typical marijuana effects; fears of losing control produce severe anxiety.	Regular use over time may result in a loss of motivation and in the inability to handle one's responsibilities. This often results in problems in school, on the job, or in personal relationships. Although these same problems can result from regular use of many drugs, they seem to be of particular concern with marijuana. Long-term smoking of marijuana can damage the lungs and respiratory system. It can be particularly harmful because users typically inhale unfiltered smoke deeply and hold it in their lungs for long periods. Marijuana smoke contains carcinogens and ingredients that cause emphysema and block the lungs' small air passages. Because cigarette smoking also causes heart and lung diseases, including lung cancer, combining marijuana and cigarette smoking creates increased health risks. Because marijuana use can significantly increase the heart rate (up to 50% above normal), it is particularly dangerous for people with high blood pressure or heart problems.	As with tobacco use, the short- and long-term effects of smoking marijuana give athletes little or nothing to gain and much to lose. The endurance implications of the cardiorespiratory effect of smoking marijuana, coupled with the possible loss of motivation, may dissuade athletes concerned about their performance from using marijuana. Consistent with this reasoning, athletes are less likely to use marijuana than nonathletes.
Initially, opiates stimulate the higher centers of the brain and slow down the activity of the central nervous system. After the injection of a street preparation, the user feels a rush (a strong sense of pleasure) which leads to a state of contentment. In some users, the amount needed to produce this effect may also initially cause nausea and restlessness. Higher doses may cause a sensation of warmth, heaviness in the hands and feet, and a dry mouth. The user may alternate between drowsiness and being wakeful.	Regular use over time may cause infections to heart valves and linings, abscesses of the skin, and lung congestion. Unsterile solutions, syringes, and needles can also cause a variety of infections, including tetanus, liver disease, hepatitis, and HIV/AIDS. Harmful health consequences are also caused by using too much of the drug, contamination of the drug, or combining the drug with other substances.	Athletes may use opiates for pain reduction or the initial rush. However, it is not likely that athletes would use opiates in an attempt to improve performance. They are likely to use opiates for the same reasons and in the same ways as nonathletes.

Drug name	What is it?	How is it used?
Opiates *(continued)*		
Phencyclidine	Phencyclidine (PCP) is often referred to as "angel dust." It is similar to some stimulants, but it also slows down bodily functions and has pain-killing effects. It was first developed as an anesthetic, but use was restricted because of undesirable side effects. It is available as a pure, white, crystal-like powder, a tablet, or a capsule. It is easily manufactured. In powder form it often consists of 50-100% PCP. Purity and dosage levels of the drug vary widely because it is made illegally. It is often sold as mescaline, THC, or other drugs because of PCP's bad reputation.	PCP can be sniffed, smoked, swallowed, or injected. PCP is sometimes sprinkled on marijuana or parsley and smoked.
Smokeless Tobacco	Made from tobacco plants, smokeless tobacco products include chew, dip, or snuff. These products are sometimes called "spit tobacco" because their use increases saliva production, causing the user to spit. All tobacco products contain nicotine and tars.	Smokeless tobacco is usually "chewed" or "dipped" in the mouth by placing the tobacco between the lip and gums. Compounds in the tobacco are absorbed into the bloodstream. Finely ground snuff may also be inhaled through the nose into the lungs.

Short-term effects	Long-term effects and other health risks	Connection to athletics
Very large doses cause sleep; constricted pupils; moist, cold, or bluish skin; and a slowed breathing rate which may result in death.		
The effects depend on the dosage level. Increased heart rate and blood pressure, sweating, flushing, and dizziness are some possible physical responses. Higher doses may cause drowsiness, convulsions, and coma. It is difficult for users to predict or describe the drug's effects. It may change how the user experiences the body and its surroundings. Speech, vision, and muscle coordination are affected. Touch and pain are dulled. Body movements are slowed. Time is "spaced out."	Regular PCP use may have an effect on memory, perception, concentration, and judgment. Regular users may show signs of paranoia, fearfulness, and anxiety. This may lead to aggressiveness or withdrawal, including difficulty communicating. A temporary disturbance of the user's thought processes may last for days or weeks. Chronic users of PCP may experience memory and speech difficulties, as well as hearing voices that do not exist. Poisonous levels of PCP can result in death due to repeated convulsions, heart and lung failure, and broken blood vessels in the brain. However, more people die from the results of behavior produced by PCP than the drug's direct effect on the body. PCP can produce impulsive, aggressive, and violent behavior in people who do not normally exhibit this type of behavior. This behavior can lead to death from drowning, burns, falls, or motor-vehicle accidents. Users are at risk for negative effects because purity and dosage levels of the drug vary widely, and PCP may be sold as other drugs.	The general effects of PCP would not seem to lend themselves to any particular athletic use. Athletes are most likely to use these drugs for the same reasons other users would.
Nicotine stimulates the heart and central nervous system. It increases heart rate, narrows blood vessels, and elevates blood pressure. It also dilates the pupils and increases the production of saliva, which usually results in frequent spitting. Some of these effects of nicotine can result in	Extreme amounts of nicotine depress the central nervous system and may lead to death. Tars irritate many of the tissues in the body. They contain many carcinogens. Regular users of smokeless tobacco generally consume more of these tars than do regular smokers.	There is little or no basis for smokeless tobacco to have a positive effect on athletic performance. However, some athletes may perceive a positive effect, much like a certain routine that the athlete may follow before shooting a free throw or while consuming a pregame

Drug name	What is it?	How is it used?
Smokeless Tobacco *(continued)*		
Steroids (anabolic-androgenic)	Anabolic-androgenic steroids are the steroids used by individuals in an effort to gain size and strength. Anabolic refers to the constructive or building-up process of the body's metabolism. Androgenic refers to male-like or masculinizing characteristics. The steroids used in the effort to build up oneself are chemical derivatives of the male sex hormones, thus the term anabolic-androgenic. In addition to androgenic steroids, two other categories are estrogenic and corticosteroids. Estrogenic steroids produce female or feminizing characteristics. Corticosteroids are those from the cortex of the adrenal glands. They have a shrinking, not a building up, effect and are used to treat tissue stress, reduce inflammation, and ease pain.	Anabolic-androgenic steroids are either taken orally (pills or capsules) or injected with a syringe (as a viscous liquid). To build size, strength, and speed, athletes often use 10 to 100 times the medical dosage. Steroid users often cycle (go on and off) and stack (use more than one type of) steroids in attempts to maximize strength gains, minimize side effects, and avoid detection.

Short-term effects	Long-term effects and other health risks	Connection to athletics
the smokeless tobacco user feeling a "buzz." Dizziness and nausea can result from chewing or dipping tobacco, especially if the tobacco juice is swallowed. Larger amounts of nicotine may cause rapid breathing, tremors, and a decrease in urine production.	Chewing or dipping tobacco can irritate the lips, gums, throat, and stomach. It can lead to cancer in these areas. White patches can form in the mouth. These patches, called leukoplakia, can lead to cancer. The constant irritation can also cause dental problems. Chewing or dipping tobacco often leads to a decrease in the sensations of taste and smell. Smokeless tobacco users may increase the amount of sugar and salt they use on their food to improve the taste. This can contribute to an increase in blood pressure and, possibly, weight.	meal; some athletes may believe chewing enhances their performance. Marketing of smokeless tobacco to athletes may help promote two beliefs: that smokeless-tobacco use is consistent with the image of the sport and that smokeless-tobacco use is healthier than smoking. There appears to be a strong association between smokeless-tobacco use and athletes in particular sports (for example, baseball and football). Yet, young athletes may be less likely to use smokeless tobacco during their season of play.
Because steroids increase the amount of similarly existing hormones in the body, the user will likely notice few or no effects immediately after ingesting or injecting anabolic steroids. An increase in appetite, energy, or aggressiveness, and more rapid recovery from strenuous workouts may be some of the first effects noticed by steroid users, but these effects will probably not be experienced after a single dose.	Anabolic-androgenic steroid use can affect the liver and the cardiovascular system as well as the reproductive system. Liver function can be damaged, resulting in jaundice, blood-filled cysts, and tumors (including those that are cancerous). Blood cholesterol levels often increase because steroid use changes how sugars and fats are handled. This and increased blood pressure can lead to the early development of heart disease, which can increase the risk of heart attacks and strokes. For males, their production of their naturally occurring hormones, like testosterone, may be decreased. This may result in shrinking of the testes, low sperm counts, and infertility. Because anabolic-androgenic steroids are derivative of male hormones, female users may take on more male-like characteristics, such as broader backs, wider shoulders, thicker waists, flatter chests, more body and facial hair, and deeper voices. The clitoris may enlarge, and menstrual cycles may become irregular or stop.	In sports where size, strength, and speed are important factors, athletes may use anabolic steroids in an attempt to enhance these factors, characteristics, or abilities. Chapter 2 discussed some of the thinking that fuels an athlete's choice to use steroids. Athletic performance and appearance are the two most common reasons given for using anabolic-androgenic steroids (Buckley et al., 1988).

Drug name	What is it?	How is it used?
Steroids (anabolic-androgenic) *(continued)*		
Tobacco (smoking)	A wide variety of tobacco products in smoking form are made from tobacco plants. These products include cigarettes, cigars, and pipe tobacco. All tobacco products contain nicotine and tars. In addition, carbon monoxide is produced in the smoking process.	Cigarettes, cigars, and pipe tobacco are smoked and inhaled into the lungs.

Short-term effects	Long-term effects and other health risks	Connection to athletics
	Anabolic-androgenic steroids may not only affect muscles but other parts of the musculoskeletal system. Tendons and ligaments may not strengthen at the same rate the muscle tissue develops (or steroids may actually impair the strength and integrity of tendons and ligaments). As a result, these tissues appear to be injured more often among steroid users. Also, for adolescent athletes, steroid use may cause the growth plates in long bones to close faster than usual, which can result in lower height. Oily skin and acne are also common among steroid users. Some steroid users experience dramatic mood swings. Anxiety, irritability, aggressiveness, and impulsiveness may occur.	
Nicotine stimulates the heart and central nervous system. It increases heart rate, narrows blood vessels, and elevates blood pressure. It also dilates the pupils, irritates lung tissue, and increases the production of saliva. Larger amounts of nicotine may cause rapid breathing, tremors, and a decrease in urine production. Carbon monoxide inhaled into the lungs competes with oxygen to be carried by the blood. Thus, the blood's ability to carry oxygen to the body tissues is reduced. Smokers may experience shortness of breath while performing activities.	Extreme amounts of nicotine depress the central nervous system and may lead to death. Tars are irritants to many of the tissues in the body. They contain many carcinogens and have been linked to many types of cancer, most notably cancer of the lungs. Over time, smokers can develop heart and respiratory problems, including nagging coughs, chronic bronchitis, emphysema, heart disease, and lung and other types of cancer. Nonsmokers exposed to second-hand smoke may experience irritation of the eyes, nose, and throat, headaches, and other allergic reactions. Individuals with chronic heart and lung disease are very vulnerable to second-hand smoke.	Both the short- and long-term effects of smoking tobacco on the cardiorespiratory system could affect an athlete's endurance. Most athletes recognize that there is little or nothing to gain and much to lose by smoking. Consistent with this reasoning, athletes are less likely to smoke than nonathletes.

Drug name	What is it?	How is it used?
Major tranquilizers (sedative hypnotic)	Major tranquilizers come in tablets, capsules, or liquids. They are used to treat psychiatric problems because major tranquilizers calm without inducing sleep. They are also used for preventing radiation sickness, preventing nausea after surgery, and providing relief of chronic itching on the skin.	Major tranquilizers are usually obtained by a doctor's prescription. Tablets and capsules are taken by mouth.
Tricyclic Antidepressants (sedative hypnotic)	Tricyclic antidepressants or mood elevators are pills given to relieve mental depression. Amitriptyline and desipramine are two well known antidepressants.	Tricyclic antidepressants are medically prescribed and taken orally to relieve mental depression.

Short-term effects	Long-term effects and other health risks	Connection to athletics
In moderate doses, major tranquilizers produce a calming effect without inducing sleep. Low doses produce drowsiness, and high doses may produce a stupor and impair coordination. Blood pressure usually goes down while the heart rate may go up.	Almost all organ systems can be adversely affected by phenothiazines. Because most adverse reactions are related to dosage and length of use, a physician monitors use of these drugs. One of the better known side effects is tardive dyskinesia.	This category of drugs is rarely abused by anyone because of the drugs' unpleasant side effects. The category is listed here because it is possible that an athlete may use major tranquilizers under a doctor's care to treat psychiatric problems.
Dramatic effects from a single dose do not typically result. In therapeutic doses, depressed patients experience gradual mood improvement.	Tolerance for antidepressants does not appear to develop. If use of the drug abruptly ends, withdrawal symptoms, such as nausea and overall discomfort are possible.	Athletes are likely to use tricyclic antidepressants for the same reasons as other users.

References

Alcoholics Anonymous World Services, Inc. (1980). *Twelve steps and twelve traditions.* New York: Alcoholics Anonymous World Services, Inc.

Anderson, W.A., Albrecht, R.R., & McKeag, D.B. (1993). *Second replication of a national study of the substance use and abuse habits of college student-athletes: Final report.* East Lansing, MI: Michigan State University, College of Human Medicine. Paper presented at the meeting of the National Collegiate Athletic Association, Overland Park, KS.

Anderson, W.A., & McKeag, D.B. (1985). *The substance use and abuse habits of college student-athletes: General findings* (Research Paper No. 2). East Lansing, MI: Michigan State University, College of Human Medicine. Paper presented at the meeting of the National Collegiate Athletic Association Council Executive Committee Drug Education Committee, Mission, KS.

Anderson, W.A., & McKeag, D.B. (1989). *Replication of the national study of the substance use and abuse habits of college student-athletes: Final report.* East Lansing, MI: Michigan State University, College of Human Medicine. Paper presented at the meeting of the National Collegiate Athletic Association, Mission, KS.

Benson, P.L. (1990). *The troubled journey: A portrait of 6th-12th grade youth.* Minneapolis: Lutheran Brotherhood.

Blaszczak, S. (1992). *The parent network manual.* Apple Valley, MN: Author.

Buckley, W.E., Yesalis, C.E., Friedl, K.E., Anderson, W.A., Streit, A.L., & Wright, J.E. (1988). Estimated prevalence of anabolic steroid use among male high school seniors. *Journal of the American Medical Association,* **260**, 3441-3445.

Carr, C.M., Kennedy, S.R., & Dimick, K.M. (1990). Alcohol use among high school athletes: A comparison of alcohol use and intoxication in male and female high school athletes and non-athletes. *Journal of Alcohol and Drug Education,* **36**(1), 39-45.

Court clouds legality of student drug testing. (1994, June). *School Board News*, **14**(10), 1, 6.

Escobedo, L.G., Marcus, S.E., Holtzman, D., & Giovino, G.A. (1993). Sports participation, age at smoking initiation, and the risk of smoking among U.S. high school students. *Journal of the American Medical Association*, **269**, 1391-1395.

Extra curricular involvement. (1995, February). *Youth Update*, 3.

Funk, J., Svendsen, R., Cunningham, K., & Griffin, T.M. (1989). *Student assistance model: The response component*. Center City, MN: Hazelden.

Harding, Ringhofer & Associates, Inc. (1992). *Everyone a hero*. Aurora, CO: Colorado State High School Activities Association.

Harding, Ringhofer & Associates, Inc. (1994). *TARGET leadership training manual*. Kansas City, MO: National Federation TARGET Program.

Hawkins, J.D., & Catalano, R.F., Jr. (1992). *Communities that care: Action for drug abuse prevention*. San Francisco: Jossey-Bass.

Iowa High School Athletic Association. (1990). *Athletic participation? Students give their views* [Pamphlet]. Boone, IA: Author.

Iowa High School Athletic Association. (1993). *Suggestions for coaches and athletic directors using the "Pledge to Be Alcohol- and Drug-Free" cards* [Pamphlet]. Boone, IA: Author.

Johnston, L.D., O'Malley, P.M., & Bachman, J.G. (1993a). *National survey results on drug use from the Monitoring the Future study, 1975-1992: Secondary school students* (Vol. 1, NIH Publication No. 93-3597). Rockville, MD: National Institute on Drug Abuse.

Johnston, L.D., O'Malley, P.M., & Bachman, J.G. (1993b). *National survey results on drug use from the Monitoring the Future study, 1975-1992: College students and young adults* (Vol. 2, NIH Publication No. 93-3598). Rockville, MD: National Institute on Drug Abuse.

Johnston, L.D., O'Malley, P.M., & Bachman, J.G. (1994). *National survey results on drug use from the Monitoring the Future study, 1975-1993: Secondary school students*. (Vol. 1, NIH Publication No. 94-3809). Rockville, MD: National Institute on Drug Abuse.

Massachusetts Interscholastic Athletic Association. (1993). *The Massachusetts Interscholastic Athletic Association's rules of and regulations governing athletics: Rule #71: Chemical health* [Pamphlet]. Milford, MA: Author.

Minnesota Department of Education and Risk Reduction Unit. (1992). *Minnesota student survey, 1989-1992: Reflections of social change*. St. Paul, MN: Minnesota Department of Education.

Minnesota Prevention Resource Center. (1985). *Non-alcoholic party drinks*. Anoka, MN: Minnesota Prevention Resource Center.

Minnesota State High School League. (1990). *1990-1991 official handbook*. Brooklyn Center, MN: Author.

Minnesota State High School League. (1991). *1991-1992 athletic eligibility information* [Pamphlet]. Brooklyn Center, MN: Author.

Minnesota State High School League. (1994). *Minnesota state high school league 1994-95 eligibility information* [Pamphlet]. Brooklyn Center, MN: Author.

National Federation TARGET Program. (1991). *TARGET national coaches survey on perceptions of teenage tobacco, alcohol, and other drug use.* Kansas City, MO: Author.

National Federation TARGET Program. (1993a). *Playing fair, keeping fit, looking good without using steroids.* Presentation with the assistance of the Center for Substance Abuse Prevention Communications Team at the meeting of the National Federation TARGET Program, Kansas City, MO.

National Federation TARGET Program. (1993b). *Preseason meeting handbook.* Kansas City, MO: Author.

Nattiv, A., & Puffer, J.C. (1991). Lifestyles and health risks of collegiate athletes. *The Journal of Family Practice,* **33,** 585-590.

Ringhofer, K., & Harding, M. (1993). *When is when?* [Pamphlet]. Minnetonka, MN: Harding, Ringhofer & Associates, Inc.

Skolnick, A.A. (1993). Studies raise doubts about benefit of athletics in reducing unhealthy behavior among adolescents. *Journal of the American Medical Association,* **270,** 798-799.

Substance Abuse and Mental Health Services Administration Office of Applied Studies. (1993). *National household survey on drug abuse: Population estimates 1992.* (DHHS Publication No. SMA 93-2053). Rockville, MD: U.S. Department of Health and Human Services.

Svendsen, R., & Griffin, T. (1990). *Choosing not to use alcohol: Benefits for adolescents* [Pamphlet]. Sturgis, MI: Ruster Foundation.

Svendsen, R., & Harding, M. (1987). *A preseason meeting: A guide for parents in responding to alcohol and other drug issues.* Kansas City, MO: TARGET.

U.S. Department of Agriculture and U.S. Department of Health and Human Services. (1991, September/October). Dietary guidelines for Americans. *Prevention Pipeline,* **4**(5), 68.

U.S. Department of Health and Human Services. (1993). *National household survey on drug abuse: Population estimates 1992.* Rockville, MD: Substance Abuse and Mental Health Services Administration, Office of Applied Studies.

U.S. Department of Health and Human Services. (1994). *Preventing tobacco use among young people: A report of the surgeon general.* Atlanta, GA: U.S. Deparment of Health and Human Services, Public Health Service, Centers for Disease Control and Prevention, National Center for Chronic Disease Prevention and Health Promotion, Office on Smoking and Health.

Wallack, L., Cassady, D., & Grube, J. (1990). *TV, beer commercials, and children: Exposure, attention, beliefs, and expectations about drinking as an adult.* Washington, DC: AAA Foundation for Traffic Safety.

Index

About the Authors

Kevin R. Ringhofer and Martha E. Harding are codirectors of Harding, Ringhofer & Associates, Inc. (HRA), an organization that educates coaches, school staff members, student leaders, and parents about how to prevent tobacco, alcohol, and other drug use among students. They are also consultants for the National Federation of State High School Associations TARGET healthy lifestyles program.

Kevin and Martha have worked with TARGET and other organizations to develop and moderate three national satellite teleconferences: *The Spitting Image*, which focused on preventing the use of smokeless tobacco; *Everybody's Business*, which provided prevention training for teachers, coaches, and other youth workers; and *HIV and Sports: Understanding Our Responsibility*, which explored the role of sports organizations in preventing the transmission of HIV/AIDS and other blood-borne pathogens.

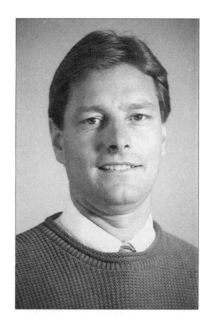

Kevin earned a PhD in physical education from the University of Minnesota in 1991. Before working at HRA, Kevin was program supervisor of the Hazelden-Cork Sports Education Program and project and research assistant at the University of Minnesota. He has provided training and technical assistance to schools, businesses, and other community organizations on such topics as tobacco, alcohol, and other drug-use issues; physical activity and fitness; and stress management. In his leisure time, Kevin enjoys playing softball and baseball, biking, and participating in church youth group activities.

Martha, who has a BA in English and education from Augsburg College in Minneapolis, has worked in health and human services for more than 20 years. Before becoming codirector of HRA she was a national trainer and consultant in prevention and health promotion for the Hazelden Foundation. She has developed several cross-age education and mentoring programs that encourage high school athletes to send positive nonuse messages to younger students. Martha is a member of the National Association of Prevention Professionals and Advocates, the Community Partnership with Youth and Families, and the Minnesota Prevention Network. In her spare time, Martha enjoys hiking, camping, biking, music, and drama.

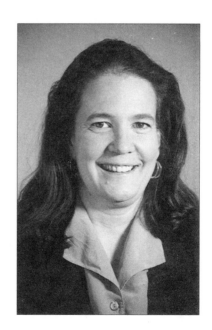

The Coaching Successfully Series

The books in the Coaching Successfully Series explain how to teach fundamental sports skills and strategies as well as how to apply principles of philosophy, psychology, and teaching and management methods to coaching. Each sport-specific book shows you not only what to teach athletes but also how to teach it.

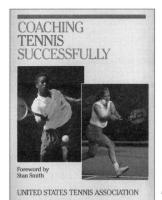

Coaching Tennis Successfully

United States Tennis Association

Foreword by Stan Smith

1995 • Paper • 200 pp
Item PUST0461
ISBN 0-87322-461-2
$18.95 ($26.50 Canadian)

"I cannot imagine a better all-around book for setting up an entire tennis program. A must for all tennis coaches."

Bob Wood
Executive Committee, National High School Athletic Coaches Association

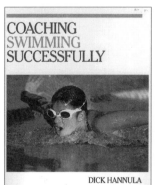

Coaching Swimming Successfully

Dick Hannula

Foreword by Skip Kenney

1995 • Paper • 176 pp
Item PHAN0492
ISBN 0-87322-492-2
$18.95 ($26.50 Canadian)

"Organized and succinct, this book will benefit all coaches who read and study it."

Peter Daland, President, American Swim Coaches Association; Former USC Head Men's Swimming Coach

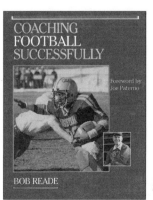

Coaching Football Successfully

Bob Reade

Foreword by Joe Paterno

1994 • Paper • 192 pp
Item PREA0518
ISBN0-87322-518-X
$18.95 ($27.95 Canadian)

"This book should be the bible of how to coach and lead young men on every level of football."

Hayden Fry
Head Football Coach
The University of Iowa

Coaching Basketball Successfully

Morgan Wootten

Foreword by John Wooden

1992 • Paper • 240 pp
Item PWOO0446
ISBN 0-88011-446-0
$18.95 ($26.50 Canadian)

"This is the most comprehensive basketball book that I have read."

Rick Pitino
Head Basketball Coach
University of Kentucky

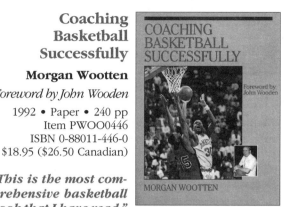

Coaching Volleyball Successfully

William J. Neville, BS, USA Volleyball (formerly US Volleyball Association)

1990 • Paper • 224 pp
Item PNEV0362
ISBN 0-88011-362-6
$18.00 ($24.95 Canadian)

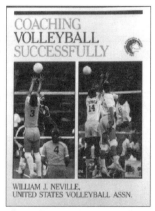

Coaching Girls' Basketball Successfully

Jill Hutchison, EdD, in cooperation with the Women's Basketball Coaches Association

1989 • Paper • 288 pp
Item PHUT0343
ISBN 0-88011-343-X
$20.00 ($27.95 Canadian)

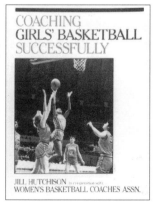

Human Kinetics
The Premier Publisher for Sports & Fitness

Prices are subject to change.

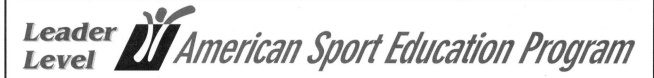
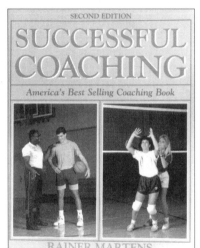
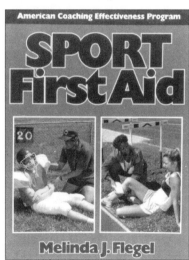
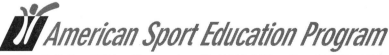